T0321080

INTERVENTIONAL CARDIOLOGY CLINICS

www.interventional.theclinics.com

Editor-in-Chief

MARVIN H. ENG

STATE OF THE ART IN STEMI CARE

July 2021 • Volume 10 • Number 3

Editor

RAVI S. HIRA

ELSEVIER

1600 John F. Kennedy Boulevard • Suite 1800 • Philadelphia, Pennsylvania, 19103-2899

http://www.theclinics.com

INTERVENTIONAL CARDIOLOGY CLINICS Volume 10, Number 3
July 2021 ISSN 2211-7458, ISBN-13: 978-0-323-81383-9

Editor: Joanna Collett
Developmental Editor: Arlene B. Campos

Interventional Cardiology Clinics (ISSN 2211-7458) is published quarterly by Elsevier Inc., 360 Park Avenue South, New York, NY 10010-1710. Months of issue are January, April, July, and October. Subscription prices are USD 209 per year for US individuals, USD 622 for US institutions, USD 100 per year for US students, USD 209 per year for Canadian individuals, USD 638 for Canadian institutions, USD 100 per year for Canadian students, USD 296 per year for international individuals, USD 638 for international institutions, and USD 150 per year for international students. To receive student/resident rate, orders must be accompanied by name of affiliated institution, date of term, and the *signature* of program/residency coordinator on institution letterhead. Orders will be billed at individual rate until proof of status is received. Foreign air speed delivery is included in all *Clinics* subscription prices. All prices are subject to change without notice. **POSTMASTER:** Send address changes to *Interventional Cardiology Clinics*, Elsevier Health Sciences Division, Subscription Customer Service, 3251 Riverport Lane, Maryland Heights, MO 63043. **Customer Service: Telephone: 1-800-654-2452** (U.S. and Canada); **1-314-447-8871** (outside U.S. and Canada). **Fax: 1-314-447-8029. E-mail: journalscustomerservice-usa@elsevier.com (for print support); journalsonlinesupport-usa@elsevier.com (for online support).**

Reprints. For copies of 100 or more of articles in this publication, please contact the Commercial Reprints Department, Elsevier Inc., 360 Park Avenue South, New York, NY 10010-1710. Tel.: 212-633-3874; Fax: 212-633-3820; E-mail: reprints@elsevier.com.

CONTRIBUTORS

EDITOR-IN-CHIEF

MARVIN H. ENG, MD
Structural Heart Disease Fellowship Director,
Center for Structural Heart Disease, Henry
Ford Hospital, Detroit, Michigan, USA

EDITOR

RAVI S. HIRA, MD
Pulse Heart Institute, Tacoma, Washington,
USA; Cardiac Care Outcomes Assessment
Program, Foundation for Health Care Quality,
Seattle, Washington, USA

AUTHORS

J. DAWN ABBOTT, MD
Lifespan Cardiovascular Institute, Rhode
Island Hospital, Warren Alpert Medical School
at Brown University, Providence, Rhode
Island, USA

ZIAD A. ALI, MD, DPhil
St. Francis Hospital–The Heart Center, Roslyn,
New York, USA; Clinical Trials Center,
Cardiovascular Research Foundation,
NewYork-Presbyterian Hospital/Columbia
University Irving Medical Center, New York,
New York, USA

JOE AOUN, MD
Department of Cardiovascular Medicine,
Houston Methodist DeBakey Heart & Vascular
Center, Houston, Texas, USA

JASON A. BARTOS, MD, PhD
Cardiovascular Division, Center for
Resuscitation Medicine, University of
Minnesota Medical School, University of
Minnesota, Minneapolis, Minnesota, USA

MIR B. BASIR, DO
Director, STEMI, Director, Acute Mechanical
Circulatory Support, Interventional Cardiology,
Senior Staff, Henry Ford Hospital, Henry Ford
Health Care System, Detroit, Michigan, USA

CHIRAG BAVISHI, MD, MPH
Lifespan Cardiovascular Institute, Rhode
Island Hospital, Warren Alpert Medical School

at Brown University, Providence, Rhode
Island, USA

**SONYA N. BURGESS, MBChB, PhD,
FRACP, FCSANZ, SCAI-ELM**
Academic Interventional Cardiologist,
Department of Cardiology, University of Sydney
and Nepean Hospital, University of New South
Wales, Sydney, New South Wales, Australia

JACOB A. DOLL, MD
Division of Cardiology, Department of
Medicine, University of Washington, VA Puget
Sound Health Care System, Seattle,
Washington, USA

MATTHEW C. EVANS, MD
Division of Cardiology, Medical University of
South Carolina, Charleston, South Carolina,
USA

BRITTANY FULLER, MD
Henry Ford Health Care System, Detroit,
Michigan, USA

KEYVAN KARIMI GALOUGAHI, MD, PhD
Royal Prince Alfred Hospital, University of
Sydney, Heart Research Institute, Sydney,
Australia

SACHIN S. GOEL, MD
Department of Cardiovascular Medicine,
Houston Methodist DeBakey Heart & Vascular
Center, Houston, Texas, USA

ALAYN GOVEA, MD
Cardiology Fellow, Division of Cardiovascular
Medicine, UC San Diego, San Diego, California,
USA; UC San Diego Sulpizio Cardiovascular
Center, La Jolla, California, USA

JOSHUA HAHN, MD
Section of Cardiology, Baylor College of
Medicine, Houston, Texas, USA

ALLEN JEREMIAS, MD, MSc
St. Francis Hospital–The Heart Center, Roslyn,
New York, USA

PRAJITH JEYAPRAKASH, BMed, MD,
MMed
Advanced Trainee, Department of Cardiology,
University of Sydney and Nepean Hospital,
Kingswood, New South Wales, Australia

HANI JNEID, MD, FACC, FAHA, FSCAI
Section of Cardiology, Baylor College of
Medicine, Associate Professor of Medicine,
Director, Interventional Cardiology Fellowship
Program, Director, Interventional Cardiology
Research, Baylor College of Medicine,
Director, Interventional Cardiology, The
Michael E. DeBakey VA Medical Center,
Houston, Texas, USA

TARA L. JONES, MD, PharmD
Division of Cardiovascular Medicine,
University of Utah, Salt Lake City, Utah, USA

WALEED KAYANI, MD
Section of Cardiology, Baylor College of
Medicine, Houston, Texas, USA

NEAL S. KLEIMAN, MD
Department of Cardiovascular Medicine,
Houston Methodist DeBakey Heart & Vascular
Center, Houston, Texas, USA

MARINOS KOSMOPOULOS, MD
Cardiovascular Division, Center for
Resuscitation Medicine, University of
Minnesota Medical School, University of
Minnesota, Minneapolis, Minnesota, USA

CHAYAKRIT KRITTANAWONG, MD
Section of Cardiology, Baylor College of
Medicine, Houston, Texas, USA

KATHERINE J. KUNKEL, MD, MSEd
Henry Ford Health Care System, Detroit,
Michigan, USA

JERRY LIPINKSI, MD
UC San Diego Sulpizio Cardiovascular Center,
La Jolla, California, USA; Internal Medicine
Resident, Department of Internal Medicine,
UC San Diego, San Diego, California, USA

AKIKO MAEHARA, MD
St. Francis Hospital–The Heart Center, Roslyn,
New York, USA; Clinical Trials Center,
Cardiovascular Research Foundation,
NewYork-Presbyterian Hospital/Columbia
University Irving Medical Center, New York,
New York, USA

ANBUKARASI MARAN, MD
Division of Cardiology, Medical University of
South Carolina, Charleston, South Carolina,
USA

GARY S. MINTZ, MD
Clinical Trials Center, Cardiovascular Research
Foundation, New York, New York, USA

DAN D. NGUYEN, MD
Division of Cardiology, Department of
Medicine, University of Washington, Seattle,
Washington, USA

MITUL P. PATEL, MD, FACC, FSCAI
UC San Diego Sulpizio Cardiovascular Center,
La Jolla, California, USA; Clinical Professor of
Medicine, Division of Cardiovascular
Medicine, UC San Diego Cardiovascular
Institute, San Diego, California, USA

GREGORY PETROSSIAN, BS
St. Francis Hospital–The Heart Center, Roslyn,
New York, USA

ROOPA SALWAN, MD, DM (Cardiology),
MHCD 2012 HBS
Senior Director Max MI Program, Max Super
Speciality Hospital, New Delhi, India

ASHOK SETH, FRCP, FACC, MSCAI, FESC,
FAPSIC, DSc
President, Asian Pacific Society of
Interventional Cardiology, Chairman, Fortis
Escorts Heart Institute, New Delhi, India

RASHMEE U. SHAH, MD, MS
Division of Cardiovascular Medicine,
University of Utah, Salt Lake City, Utah, USA

EVAN SHLOFMITZ, DO
St. Francis Hospital–The Heart Center, Roslyn,
New York, USA

RICHARD SHLOFMITZ, MD
St. Francis Hospital–The Heart Center, Roslyn, New York, USA

SHANTHOSH SIVAPATHAN, MBBS, MPH
Advanced Trainee, Department of Cardiology, University of Sydney and Nepean Hospital, Kingswood, New South Wales, Australia

ROBERT C. STURM, MD
Division of Cardiovascular Medicine, University of Utah, Salt Lake City, Utah, USA

DEMETRIS YANNOPOULOS, MD
Professor, Cardiovascular Division, Center for Resuscitation Medicine, University of Minnesota Medical School, University of Minnesota, Minneapolis, Minnesota, USA

SCOTT T. YOUNGQUIST, MD, MS
Division of Emergency Medicine, University of Utah, Salt Lake City, Utah, USA

SARAH J. ZAMAN, MBBS, PhD, FRACP, FCSANZ, SCAI-ELM
Associate Professor, Academic Interventional Cardiologist, Department of Cardiology, University of Sydney and Westmead Hospital, Monash University, Westmead, Australia

CONTENTS

ST-segment elevation myocardial infarction is a medical emergency with significant health care delivery challenges to ensure rapid triage and treatment. Several developments over the past decades have led to improved care delivery, decreased time to reperfusion, and decreased mortality. Still, significant challenges remain to further optimize the delivery of care for this patient population.

ST elevation myocardial infarction diagnoses have reduced in number over the past 10 years; however, associated morbidity and mortality remain high. Societal guidelines focus on early diagnosis and timely access to reperfusion, preferably percutaneous coronary intervention (PCI), with fibrinolytics reserved for those who cannot receive timely PCI. Proposed algorithms recommend emergency department bypass in stable patients with a clear diagnosis to reduced door-to-balloon time. Emergency providers should limit their evaluation, focusing on life-threatening comorbidities, unstable vitals, or contraindications to a catheterization laboratory. In-hospital patients prove diagnostically challenging because they may be unable to express symptoms, and reperfusion strategies can complicate other diagnoses.

Intravenous anticoagulation is standard of care in the treatment of ST-elevation myocardial infarction. Primary percutaneous coronary intervention is the most common reperfusion strategy. Four anticoagulant options are available: unfractionated heparin, enoxaparin, fondaparinux, and bivalirudin. This article discusses the mechanism of action and key pharmacodynamic characteristics of these agents. The evolution of outcomes with unfractionated heparin compared with bivalirudin in the changing landscape of contemporary percutaneous coronary intervention is chronicled. Current anticoagulation recommendations from practice guidelines are provided and unresolved issues including treatment of patient subsets such as women and chronic kidney disease are explored.

Distal embolization of thrombus can lead to impairment of microvascular perfusion, and measures of abnormal microvascular perfusion have been associated with increased mortality and worsened clinical outcomes. Large multicenter randomized controlled trials and multiple meta-analyses have failed to demonstrate an improvement in clinical outcomes with the routine use of manual aspiration thrombectomy, with some studies suggesting an increased incidence of stroke, likely owing to thrombus dislodgement during retrieval leading to cerebral vessel embolization. In patients with high thrombus burden who do not respond to balloon predilation, the use of manual aspiration thrombectomy as a bailout treatment strategy can be considered.

Advances in intravascular imaging have enabled assessment of the underlying plaque morphology in acute coronary syndromes, which allows for the initiation of individualized therapy. The atherothrombotic substrates for acute coronary syndromes consist of plaque rupture, erosion, and calcified nodule, whereas spontaneous coronary artery dissection, coronary artery spasm, and coronary embolism constitute rarer nonatherothrombotic etiologies. This review provides a brief overview of the data from clinical studies that have used intravascular optical coherence tomography to assess the culprit plaque morphology. We discuss the usefulness of intravascular imaging for effective treatment of patients presenting with acute coronary syndromes by percutaneous coronary intervention.

For decades, advances in ST elevation myocardial infarction (STEMI) care have been driven by timely reperfusion of the occluded culprit vessel. More recently, however, the focus has shifted to revascularization of nonculprit vessels in STEMI patients. Five landmark randomized trials, all published in the past 7 years, have highlighted the importance of complete revascularization in STEMI treatment. This review focuses on evidence-based management of STEMI in the setting of multivessel disease, highlighting contemporary data that investigate the impact of complete revascularization.

Acute myocardial infarction and cardiogenic shock (AMI-CS) is associated with significant morbidity and mortality. Early mechanical revascularization improves survival, and development of STEMI systems of care has increased the utilization of revascularization in AMI-CS from 19% in 2001 to 60% in 2014. Mechanical circulatory support devices are increasingly used to support and prevent hemodynamic collapse. These devices provide different levels of univentricular and biventricular support, have different mechanisms of actions, and provide different physiologic effects. Herein, the authors review the definition, incidence, pathophysiology, and treatment of AMI-CS.

evidence for quality improvement interventions along the spectrum of STEMI care, describes existing systems for quality measurement, and examines local and national policy interventions, with special attention to public reporting programs.

Development of ST-elevation Myocardial Infarction Programs in Developing Countries: Global Challenges and Solutions

Roopa Salwan and Ashok Seth

Cardiovascular disease (CVD) is the leading cause of death worldwide; approximately 80% of CVD deaths occur in low-income and middle-income countries (LMICs). The epidemiologic transition to a high burden of ischemic heart disease (IHD) has happened with greater rapidity in LMICs than in high-income countries. The absolute number of individuals with premature IHD has increased substantially. Higher event rates are observed compared with high-income countries. The technological capability to do extraordinary things for patients has increased, as has patient demand, in a setting of constrained resources and expensive health care of variable quality.

STATE OF THE ART IN STEMI CARE

FOREWORD

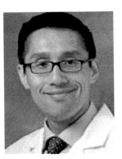

Marvin H. Eng, MD
Consulting Editor

We are pleased to introduce this issue of *Interventional Cardiology Clinics* discussing the state-of-the-art in ST-segment elevation myocardial infarction (STEMI). These patients present with a broad spectrum of clinical syndromes and sometimes have the highest acuity in the hospital. A major challenge in STEMI care is the time-sensitive relationship between treatment and outcomes, making STEMI as much a logistical as a technical and clinical management challenge.

Progress in STEMI management like most things is multifaceted. Keys to improvement in outcomes include patient's care systems, pharmacology, technical expertise, and postprocedural care. Given that the "chain of survival" involves so many providers, from emergency medical technicians, emergency room medical personnel to the interventional cardiologists, all need to coalesce together toward a common goal that is time and teamwork intensive. Aggressive pharmacologic agents have been refined in the past decade, and while STEMI cases can be the most hypercoagulable cases, care must be taken to avoid bleeding, an especially morbid scenario combined with a procoagulable state. A fraction of the patients degenerate into cardiogenic shock and presents as an intense clinical dilemma. Reperfusion, pharmacology, hemodynamics, and use of mechanical circulatory support make STEMI-related cardiogenic shock one of the most challenging emergencies in medicine.

This issue of *Interventional Cardiology Clinics* has been edited by Dr Ravi S. Hira, an expert in treating coronary artery disease. We congratulate Dr Hira for assembling a comprehensive issue covering the entire gamut of issues associated with STEMI management. Readers should find this a valuable resource for improving STEMI care.

Marvin H. Eng, MD
Center for Structural Heart Disease
Henry Ford Hospital
2799 West Grand Boulevard
Clara Ford Pavilion RM 434
Detroit, MI 48202, USA

E-mail address:
Meng1@hfhs.org

Intervent Cardiol Clin 10 (2021) xiii
https://doi.org/10.1016/j.iccl.2021.04.002
2211-7458/21/© 2021 Published by Elsevier Inc.

PREFACE

Contemporary Management of Patients with ST Elevation Myocardial Infarction

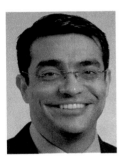

Ravi S. Hira, MD
Editor

Management of patients with acute myocardial infarction (MI) and ST elevation myocardial infarction (STEMI) has changed dramatically over the last 50 years. Recent trials have further added to our understanding since the last issue of this publication in 2016. I am thankful to all the authors that have contributed to this issue to update us on all aspects of STEMI care.

We begin with an understanding of regional systems of care and how they have significantly changed over time. While much emphasis has been placed on door-to-balloon times in the past, there is now a focus on the continuum of care and decreasing first medical contact to device times with a goal of <60 minutes, which is a new metric that is being routinely tracked and improved upon. This has been made feasible with prehospital ECG, early catheterization lab activation, and Emergency Department bypass.

Antiplatelet therapy, including newer P2Y$_{12}$ drugs and intravenous cangrelor, is discussed. Recent trials, including the ISAR REACT-5, randomized STEMI patients to prasugrel versus ticagrelor and demonstrated no significant difference between groups, including with major bleeding; however, recurrent MI was higher with ticagrelor.

Regarding anticoagulation strategies, unfractionated heparin or bivalirudin, with or without use of glycoprotein inhibitors (GPI), is the most commonly used. Contemporary trials comparing the 2 anticoagulants, including the MATRIX and VALIDATE-SWEDEHEART trials, are discussed. The VALIDATE-SWEDEHEART trial included use of newer antiplatelet therapies (95% ticagrelor) and high rates of radial access (90%) with minimal GPI use and showed no difference in the primary endpoint or major bleeding between unfractionated heparin and bivalirudin in the STEMI cohort. These trials have led to decreasing enthusiasm for Bivalirudin given similar bleeding outcomes with heparin in the setting of increased rates of radial percutaneous coronary intervention (PCI) and decreased GPI use.

New data looking at aspiration thrombectomy included results of the TOTAL trial, which showed no difference in the primary composite outcome of cardiovascular death, recurrent MI, cardiogenic shock, or NYHA class IV heart failure between patients randomized to upfront aspiration thrombectomy versus PCI alone, while patients undergoing thrombectomy had a higher incidence of stroke. Based on this trial as well as others, routine use of aspiration thrombectomy in STEMI is not recommended. However, in patients with high-thrombus burden who do not respond to balloon predilatation aspiration, thrombectomy could be used as a bailout strategy.

Another area of much interest recently has been the use of intracoronary imaging, including

Intervent Cardiol Clin 10 (2021) xv–xvi
https://doi.org/10.1016/j.iccl.2021.04.004
2211-7458/21/© 2021 Published by Elsevier Inc.

intravascular ultrasound and optical coherence tomography, which have enabled better understanding of underlying plaque morphology, atherothrombotic substrates, including plaque rupture, erosion, and calcified nodules, and enabled initiation of individualized treatment. New data are presented, and trials are underway.

Perhaps the most important change in contemporary management of STEMI patients has been in patients with multivessel disease. While prior focus had been on timely revascularization of the culprit vessel, this has been shifting to revascularization of nonculprit vessels with 5 landmark trials, including the most recent COMPLETE trial showing improved long-term outcomes, including mortality, with complete revascularization in STEMI patients.

This is not the case for STEMI patients with cardiogenic shock and multivessel disease. The CULPRIT SHOCK trial, which randomized patients to culprit only versus immediate multivessel PCI, demonstrated a significant reduction in the primary outcome and 30-day mortality with the culprit-only PCI strategy and has led to significant practice change.

Furthermore, for patients with STEMI and cardiogenic shock, mechanical circulatory support devices are being increasingly used to prevent hemodynamic collapse. With intraaortic balloon pump found to have limited utility, new trials are underway to evaluate use of extracorporeal membrane oxygenation and Impella. In addition, organized shock systems and teams with algorithmic approaches have been found to improve outcomes in these sick patients.

Unfortunately, despite all the progress made with STEMI patients, late presentation occurs in 8.5% and 40% of patients. These patients are at increased risk of mechanical complications, which can be catastrophic. While randomized trials have demonstrated a benefit of revascularization in symptomatic and hemodynamically unstable late presenters, controversy still abounds in late presenters that are asymptomatic and where stress testing may help guide management.

While PCI is the primary reperfusion strategy for STEMI, fibrinolytic therapy continues to be a reasonable option in rural communities and developing countries where timely PCI may not be an option. For these situations, a pharmacoinvasive approach is currently recommended by guidelines and is the preferred strategy. It involves immediate fibrinolysis and transfer to a PCI-capable facility and early routine PCI within 3 to 24 hours. Fibrinolysis was also widely used during the early months of the COVID-19 pandemic due to operational challenges related to PCI and COVID-19 transmission.

Much has been done to widely implement evidence-based treatment and strategies for patients with STEMI. A significant win in health care in the United States and other developed countries has been the tremendous quality improvement work that has been done at local, regional, and national levels to improve care processes and patient outcomes. However, there continue to be opportunities to further minimize variation between hospitals as well as to optimize care pathways and reduce disparities in care delivery.

Furthermore, we look at the challenges and complexity of managing STEMI patients globally where approximately 80% of cardiovascular deaths occurs in low- and middle-income countries, 40% of which are in younger patients, with 3 million STEMIs per year. Globalization and urbanization have increased cardiovascular risk in these populations, and coupled with population growth, the absolute number of individuals with premature CAD has increased substantially.

In conclusion, I hope you find this publication helpful in contributing to your knowledge and caring for your patients. As you will note reading these articles, with many new trials and data now available, STEMI care has changed remarkably over the last 5 years. While a tremendous amount of hard-earned progress has been made in getting us to where we are, much work remains. I look forward to what we will learn next.

Ravi S. Hira, MD
Pulse Heart Institute
1901 South Cedar Street #301
Tacoma, WA 98405, USA

Cardiac Care Outcomes Assessment Program
Foundation for Health Care Quality
Seattle, WA, USA

E-mail address:
hira.ravi@gmail.com

Twitter: @Ravi_Hira_MD (R.S. Hira)

Regional Systems of Care in ST Elevation Myocardial Infarction

Robert C. Sturm, MD[a],*, Tara L. Jones, MD, PharmD[a],
Scott T. Youngquist, MD, MS[b],
Rashmee U. Shah, MD, MS[a]

KEYWORDS
• STEMI • Percutaneous coronary interventions • Health services research • Quality improvement

KEY POINTS
• Timely reperfusion with primary percutaneous coronary intervention (pPCI) is the preferred treatment strategy for ST-segment elevation myocardial infarction (STEMI).
• Randomized controlled trial data demonstrate that pPCI is preferred, even if patients must be transferred to percutaneous coronary intervention (PCI)-capable hospitals.
• Observational data demonstrate that delays to reperfusion (with pPCI or thrombolysis) are associated with increased mortality among STEMI patients.
• Regional systems of care involve emergency medical services, non–PCI-capable referring hospitals, and PCI-capable STEMI receiving centers. These systems have reduced time to reperfusion with associated mortality improvements in STEMI.

INTRODUCTION

ST-segment elevation myocardial infarction (STEMI) is a medical emergency that requires immediate diagnosis and prompt intervention. Rapid treatment with primary percutaneous coronary intervention (pPCI) reduces mortality,[1] but the benefit hinges on timely treatment. The consequences of delayed treatment extend beyond in-hospital adverse outcomes and mortality; untreated STEMI or delayed reperfusion results in long-term disability, including left ventricular dysfunction and chronic kidney disease.[2–4] Randomized controlled trials and quality improvement initiatives like the Door-to-Balloon Alliance and Mission: Lifeline have emphasized rapid access to pPCI in STEMI treatment, promoting performance measures to reduce the time between STEMI onset and reperfusion.[5,6] These efforts require complex care coordination and rapid access to a percutaneous coronary intervention (PCI)-capable hospital. Over the past decade, regional systems of coordinated care have evolved to meet this need.

In order to achieve rapid pPCI treatment in STEMI, emergency medical services (EMS) must coordinate with local hospitals to develop protocols for field identification of STEMI among patients who call 911, destination protocols to direct STEMI patients to the nearest STEMI receiving hospital, and prearrival notification to the receiving center. Likewise, local hospitals require internal systems to mobilize the cardiac catheterization team for PCI. At non–PCI-capable hospitals, the team must have rapid transfer agreements with regional hospitals to transfer in a timely manner. All of these require multidisciplinary care collaboration.

Prior data from the Global Registry of Acute Coronary Events demonstrated that almost one-third of STEMI patients in the United States did not receive reperfusion treatment of any

[a] Division of Cardiovascular Medicine, University of Utah, 30 N. 1900 E, Room 4A100, Salt Lake City, UT, 84132, USA; [b] Division of Emergency Medicine, University of Utah, 30 N 1900 E 1C026, Salt Lake City, UT 84132, USA
* Corresponding author.
E-mail address: Bobby.Sturm@hsc.utah.edu

Intervent Cardiol Clin 10 (2021) 281–291
https://doi.org/10.1016/j.iccl.2021.03.001

kind, and nearly one-third received thrombolytic therapy, as opposed to the preferred pPCI strategy.[7] In recent years, regional systems of STEMI care have enabled care coordination, resulting in greater reperfusion rates, shorter time to reperfusion, and improved outcomes for STEMI patients.[8–10] This article discusses the evidence that supports pPCI as the preferred STEMI treatment, utility of thrombolytic therapy in certain scenarios, postreperfusion care, and the successful regional systems for care required to implement this treatment strategy at a population level as well as remaining challenges from a health system standpoint.

DISCUSSION

Therapeutic Interventions

The concept of a ruptured plaque in the coronary artery as the cause of STEMI was established in the 1970s.[11] The feasibility of percutaneous transluminal coronary angioplasty (PTCA) to treat stenotic coronary arteries initially was demonstrated in 1977.[12] Subsequently, a series of clinical trials demonstrated the effectiveness of thrombolytic therapy with streptokinase for patients presenting with STEMI, followed by several trials demonstrating primary PTCA was superior to thrombolytic therapy for STEMI treatment.[1,13] In 1994, the Palmaz-Schatz stent proved efficacious in treatment of symptomatic coronary artery disease and led to improved procedural success with lower rates of angiographic restenosis.[14]

As PCI technology improved, the evidence evolved first to support PTCA, then PCI, as the primary, preferred treatment of STEMI. Evidence dating back to 1993 supports the use of PTCA over thrombolysis for acute myocardial infarction (AMI) with in-hospital mortality rates, respective, of 2.6% versus 6.5% ($P = .06$). A meta-analysis found mortality benefits for patients treated with PTCA or pPCI over thrombolytics (4.4% vs 6.5%, respectively; $P = .02$) as well as a favorable outcome for hemorrhagic stroke and reinfarction rates in favor of pPCI.[1] Thus, the clinical question evolved from, "Should STEMI patients receive pPCI?" to "How can a system be created such that a high proportion of STEMI patients receive pPCI?" Although STEMI patients present to all hospitals, all hospitals are not PCI-capable. The challenge is how to rapidly recognize and triage STEMI patients for pPCI, with transfer to a PCI-capable center, if feasible.

The first steps in answering this question came from 2 randomized trials. The DANAMI-2 and PRAGUE-2 trials tested the hypothesis that

pPCI (even if transfer to a PCI-capable facility from a non–PCI-capable hospital was needed) was superior to immediate thrombolysis in STEMI treatment (Table 1). PRAGUE-2 included STEMI patients who presented to non–PCI-capable hospitals in the Czech Republic, did not suffer cardiac arrest, and had no contraindications to thrombolytic therapy. These patients were randomized to receive either immediate thrombolysis or transfer to a PCI-capable hospital for pPCI. In this patient cohort, the rate of 30-day mortality was lower among patients who received pPCI compared with those who received thrombolytic therapy (6.8% vs 10%, respectively; $P = .12$ based on intention to treat analysis; 6.0% vs 10.4%, respectively; $P < .05$ based on treatment received).[15] In DANAMI-2, a similar trial conducted in Denmark, the primary outcome (a composite of death, clinical evidence of reinfarction, and disabling stroke at 30 days) occurred less often among patients randomized to pPCI compared with thrombolytic therapy (6.7% vs 12.3%, respectively; $P = .05$). This difference was driven mainly by higher rates of recurrent reinfarction among patients randomized to thrombolysis; mortality rates were similar between the 2 arms (6.6% vs 7.8%, respectively; $P = .35$).[16]

Thus, the DANAMI-2 and PRAGUE-2 trials suggested that primary PCI is preferred even if this approach requires a delay for transfer to a

Table 1
Details of two trials that established the role of regional systems of care to support primary percutaneous coronary intervention for ST-segment elevation myocardial infarction treatment

Trial	PRAGUE-2[15]	DANAMI-2[16]
Year of publication	2002	2003
Country	Czech Republic	Denmark
Number of patients	850	1572
Primary PCI	429	790
Thrombolytics	421	782
Longest distance for transfer, km (miles)	120 (75)	150 (93)
30-d mortality for PCI, %	6.8	6.6
30-d mortality for thrombolytics, %	10	7.8

PCI-capable facility, provided the transfer process and pPCI occur in a timely manner. Importantly, these studies suggested that transfer is safe. The DANAMI-2 investigators noted no deaths during the transfer process and the PRAGUE-2 investigators reported improved outcomes with pPCI, even if patient presentation was greater than 3 hours from symptom onset. No patient in PRAGUE-2 was transferred more than 120 km (approximately 75 miles) and no patient in DANAMI-2 was transferred more than 150 km (approximately 90 miles).

Early Experience with Regional Systems for ST-segment Elevation Myocardial Infarction Care in the United States

Following the results of PRAGUE-2 and DANAMI-2, efforts to implement similar infrastructure for STEMI triage and treatment began in the United States. Despite numerous, disconnected hospital systems and greater distances for travel, Henry and colleagues[17] demonstrated that such an infrastructure was feasible in the United States. Specifically, the team at the Minnesota Heart Institute followed an algorithmic approach already in place for level 1 trauma patients to facilitate rapid transfer of STEMI patients within 24 hours of symptom onset to a central, PCI-capable hospital. The referring, non–PCI-capable hospitals were grouped into 2 zones; zone 1 hospitals were within 60 miles and zone 2 hospitals were within 60 miles to 210 miles of the central hospital. All emergency department (ED) clinicians were able to activate the STEMI system with a single phone call and protocol checklists were provided to all referring facilities. The mortality outcomes of this system were favorable: among patients transferred from zone 1, the 30-day mortality rate was 4.6%, and among patients from zone 2, the 30-day mortality rate was 5.7%.

Although promising, this early experience with regional systems of STEMI care had limitations. First, the study lacked a comparison patient group who were not part of the protocol and thus could not account for simultaneous improvements in STEMI care outside of PCI (eg, rapid performance of an electrocardiogram [ECG] and early diagnosis). Inclusion of patients who were not transferred for STEMI would strengthen the results. Still, the protocol included transfer of patients up to 210 miles from the PCI-capable hospital, a large jump from the earlier randomized studies. Given the emerging consensus for pPCI as the preferred treatment of STEMI, the Minnesota experience was an important demonstration project for the feasibility of a protocol driven, regional system for STEMI patient care.

Evolution of Performance Measures: Door-to-Balloon Time

Several observational studies demonstrated a direct association between time from presentation to reperfusion and outcomes in STEMI. Thus, time to treatment became a major focus of STEMI systems of care.[18,19] Regional systems of care, like the Minnesota system, described previously, use metrics like door-to-balloon (D2B) time, door-in to door-out (DIDO) time, and first medical contact (FMC)-to-device time to evaluate success. Guidelines and performance measures provide specific goals for each of these and other metrics (Table 2).[20]

Initial performance measures focused on D2B times. Studies from the American College of Cardiology National Cardiovascular Data Registry (NCDR) indicated that longer D2B times were associated with a higher risk of in-hospital mortality. Mortality was 3.2% among patients with D2B less than or equal to 60 minutes compared with 7.7% among patients with D2B time greater than or equal to 120 minutes.[19]

In light of the emerging evidence for timely reperfusion, national organizations began to work together to create the data systems needed to develop performance measures, iteratively examine outcomes to learn and update the metrics, and inform the STEMI treatment guidelines. The Door-to-Balloon Alliance, built off the NCDR registries, sought "to achieve D2B times of 90 minutes, or less, for at least 75% of nontransfer patients receiving a pPCI" by distributing educational materials and tools, and providing hospitals with regular feedback about performance. Bradley and colleagues[5] reported increased rates of several process measures, including ED catheterization laboratory activation and prehospital laboratory activation, as well as improved D2B times among participating hospitals.

Despite these improvements, studies from the NCDR CathPCI Registry suggested that reduced D2B times alone may not have the desired effect on mortality outcomes.[21,22] These studies evaluated D2B times alone, however, and did not account for time prior to hospital arrival; the latter metric could be associated with better outcomes, particularly because the systems of care evolved to include EMS and prehospital efforts. In addition, transfer patients were excluded, which presumably included patients who transferred from one hospital's ED to another hospital's catheterization laboratory.

Table 2
Performance and quality measure goals for regional ST-segment elevation myocardial infraction systems of care

Metric	Definition	Goal
Door-to-ECG time	Among patients presenting with chest pain or other concerning symptoms, the time between patient arrival in the ED and acquisition of first ECG	<10 min
DIDO time	Among patients transferring for PCI, the time spent between arrival at a non–PCI-capable hospital and departure for PCI-capable hospital	<30 min
Door-to-needle time	Among patients with STEMI not capable of being transferred for pPCI in <120 min, the time spent between arrival and the administration of thrombolytic therapy	<30 min
D2B time	Among patients with STEMI not receiving thrombolytic therapy, the time spent between arrival at the PCI-capable hospital and angioplasty of the culprit vessel	<90 min for patients presenting to PCI-capable hospitals, <120 min for patients needing transfer to PCI-capable hospitals
FMC-to-device time	Among patients with STEMI not receiving thrombolytic therapy, the time spent between FMC (including prehospital personnel) and angioplasty of the culprit vessel	<120 min

These goals are endorsed by the ACCF/AHA and the ESC.[36,68]

Thus, these studies could obscure the impact of regional systems, particularly in regions where rural or critical access hospitals often are intermediaries.

Evolution of Performance Measures: Door-in to Door-out, First Medical Contact–to–Device, Emergency Department Bypass

Coordination of care begins before arrival at the "door" of the PCI-capable facility. Among patients who present to a non–PCI-capable hospital, the metric is not D2B time but rather first door–to–device time—the time between patient arrival at the first, non–PCI-capable hospital to PTCA at the second, PCI-capable hospital. Again, using data from the NCDR, Dauerman and colleagues23 evaluated first door–to–device time among STEMI patients who presented to non–PCI-capable hospitals but were within 60 minutes driving time of a PCI-capable hospital. Ultimately, one-third of patients evaluated in this analysis did not meet first door–to–device time of less than 120 minutes, with significant delays in DIDO times.[23] Similar findings were reported elsewhere, with additional associations between prolonged DIDO time and mortality.[24]

The Mission: Lifeline STEMI Systems Accelerator project has focused heavily on reducing FMC-to-device time and DIDO times by streamlining communication between EMS and PCI-capable hospitals.[8] Over a 1-year study period, which included approximately 23,000 patients, various regions of the country implemented an established, common protocol and training and received quarterly feedback. Via this approach, the proportion of transferred patients who received pPCI with less than 120 minutes increased from 44% to 48%.[25]

Extending the timely reperfusion concept further, American College of Cardiology Foundation (ACCF)/American Heart Association (AHA) guidelines for STEMI care updated in 2013 focused not only on D2B times but also on FMC-to-device time.[26] Using this metric, prehospital EMS time also is accounted for. Two methods to decrease prehospital time and, therefore, FMC-to-device time, include prehospital ECG acquisition and interpretation and ED bypass by EMS transport personnel. ED bypass refers to EMS personnel bypassing a closer non–PCI-capable hospital in favor of a PCI-capable hospital that may be farther away.

A report from Rokos and colleagues,[27] including multiple sites across the United States, demonstrated that prehospital ECG enabled EMS to bypass non–PCI-capable hospitals in favor of designated STEMI receiving centers, with more than 75% of patients meeting the pPCI goal D2B time of less than 90 minutes. Data from Germany demonstrate decreased mortality associated with ED bypass for stable and unstable patients, such as those with cardiogenic shock.[28] Other reports demonstrated an association between prehospital ECG/ED bypass and lower FMC-to-device times, D2B times, and STEMI mortality rates.[29–31]

Evolution of Performance Measures: Door-to-Needle

Despite growing numbers of PCI-capable centers and increasing access to pPCI, geographic imbalances continue to limit timely pPCI in some regions.[32] Nevertheless, the primary goal of timely reperfusion remains paramount to effective STEMI care and is the cornerstone for guiding the administration of thrombolytic therapy as the initial reperfusion strategy. Several studies have demonstrated a positive mortality impact with earlier administration of thrombolytic therapy when pPCI is not readily available.[33–35] Furthermore, the benefits of thrombolytic therapy are most pronounced for patients presenting within the first 12 hours of symptom onset. For clinical scenarios in which pPCI cannot reasonably be performed within 120 minutes of FMC, prompt administration of thrombolytic therapy with a goal door-to-needle time of less than or equal to 30 minutes, is recommended in the absence of contraindications, particularly if within the first 12 hours to 24 hours after symptom onset.[35] Following thrombolytic administration, patients should be transferred immediately to a PCI-capable center in the setting of cardiogenic shock, severe acute heart failure, or failed reperfusion or reocclusion. Non–PCI-capable hospitals also can consider transfer for PCI within 3 hours to 24 hours as part of a pharmacoinvasive strategy, even after successful thrombolytic therapy with stable hemodynamics.[36]

Further Growth of Regional Systems for ST-segment Elevation Myocardial Infarction Care with Focus on Performance Measures

Similar regional systems of care have been implemented elsewhere, using time metrics to evaluate success. In North Carolina, the Regional Approach to Cardiovascular Emergencies (RACE) project was implemented.[6,37] In the RACE project, a total of 119 hospitals throughout the state (21 with PCI capabilities) eventually were enrolled. Unlike in Minnesota, the RACE project did not follow a hub-and-spoke model with a central PCI-capable hospital but rather coordinated care among several hospitals with PCI capabilities across different health care systems. Specific interventions in the RACE project included the ability of paramedics or ED physicians to activate the catheterization laboratory, availability of fully staffed catheterization laboratory within 30 minutes, and regular feedback to physicians and paramedics.[6]

Although Minnesota and North Carolina represent largely rural states with few urban centers, large population centers like Los Angeles and Dallas have implemented regional systems to standardize STEMI care. In these urban settings, prompt STEMI recognition by EMS is required in order to bypass a closer, non–PCI-capable hospital in favor of direct transport to a PCI-capable hospital. In Dallas, the effort at regionalization included financial incentives to non–PCI-capable and PCI-capable hospitals as well as EMS agencies for participation. Their efforts resulted in shorter D2B over a 2-year period.[38] In Los Angeles, regionalization of STEMI care was driven by the Los Angeles County EMS Agency, which directs prehospital services for one of the country's largest municipalities both geographically and by census. Dr Bill Koenig, then medical director for Los Angeles County EMS Agency, convened a multidisciplinary council, including representatives from cardiology, emergency medicine, and EMS, to develop protocols and standards for all phases of prehospital care, along with hospital certification and reporting requirements.[39]

Similar regional systems of care, with associated impact on performance measures, are apparent outside the United States. In France, the rate of pPCI increased from 40.5% in 2005 to 76% in 2015, with corresponding declines in 6-month mortality. Although the investigators do not specify the system of care, they allude to "improved overall organization of care" and "direct admission to PCI-capable centers" as reasons for the improvement.[40] Increasing pPCI rates, shorter D2B times, and improved patient outcomes have been reported elsewhere as well.[41–43]

Patient Outcomes of Regional ST-segment Elevation Myocardial Infarction Care Systems

Although performance metrics are important, the overarching goal for regional STEMI care systems is to improve patient outcomes by reducing STEMI-related morbidity and mortality. Between 1998 and 2008, 30-day mortality rates after AMI improved from 10.5% to 7.8%. For STEMI patients, however, the mortality rate during this time remained relatively unchanged, at approximately 8% to 10%.[44,45] In addition, large studies that focus solely on D2B, as described previously, do not support impressive mortality improvements.[21,22] Although anecdotal experience suggests regional systems of care facilitate faster intervention and better outcomes, randomized or empiric observational data are needed to substantiate these efforts.

Studies and systems that focus on improving FMC-to-device time have been associated with improvements in overall STEMI mortality. Retrospective analysis of the Mission: Lifeline program, as discussed previously, demonstrated decreased in-hospital mortality by 14% at 3 years and 25% at 5 years, when adjusted for cardiac arrest. The rates of cardiogenic shock and cardiac arrest increased, however, during the observation period (2008–2012) as well as overall unadjusted mortality.[46] Similar findings were reported in 2014 study by Farshid and colleagues[47] in Australia, also with a focus on prehospital ECG.

More recent data from a German, multicenter registry suggest a positive impact of regional systems of care. FMC-to-balloon time was reduced by prehospital ECG and telephone notification prior to hospital arrival. Bypassing the ED and direct transport to the catheterization laboratory had the greatest impact, reducing FMC-to-balloon time by a mean of 33.2 minutes. FMC-to-balloon time of less than 90 minutes reduced in-hospital mortality rate to 3.9%, compared with 12.2% for FMC-to-device time, greater than 90 minutes. Similarly, an almost linear relationship was present between FMC-to-device time and mortality for STEMI patients treated within 60 minutes to 180 minutes.[48]

Postreperfusion Regional Care Systems

Approximately 8% of patients presenting with AMI develop cardiogenic shock.[49] Unfortunately, the mortality for those patients who develop cardiogenic shock following an AMI remains unacceptably high, at almost 50%.[50] Similar to the early recognition and algorithmic approach to STEMI patients, early recognition and transfer to dedicated shock centers for management of cardiogenic shock patients is paramount for optimal outcomes. Although several centers have capabilities for pPCI, only a few centers have the infrastructure, experience, and clinical

teams necessary to manage these complex shock patients, especially those needing mechanical circulatory support. In some states, such as Arizona, these dedicated acute cardiac centers are established and maintained by state law.[51]

According to the Healthcare Cost and Utilization Project National Inpatient Sample, there were approximately 10 million admissions for AMI (non-STEMI as well as STEMI) in the United States between 2000 and 2014. Of those, only 2962 were placed onto peripheral venoarterial extracorporeal membrane oxygenation (VA-ECMO). An 11-fold increase, however, in the use of VA-ECMO for these patients was observed at the end of the observation period compared with the beginning, suggesting an ever-increasing complex patient population.[52]

Although few randomized data exist to demonstrate superiority of dedicated shock centers or one mechanical support device over another, single-center experiences with dedicated shock teams have been published. For example, the University of Utah and INOVA have demonstrated statistically significant improvements for in-hospital mortality with the use of a dedicated shock team.[53,54] As more data are obtained and published, new approaches and refinements in care will develop to reduce the unacceptably high mortality rate for this patient population.

Ongoing Challenges

Regional systems of care have favorably changed the way care for STEMI patients is delivered. The end result is improved care, better outcomes, and impact on the evidence and guidelines that inform patient care. Still, STEMI patients face persistently high mortality rates and challenges remain.

First, the role of prevention in improving STEMI outcomes cannot be ignored. The return on continued improvement in D2B times and other performance metrics is limited, but there is ample room for improved primary prevention.[55]

Registries like the NCDR need to evolve to capture new data to shed light on persistently poor outcomes, while minding the participant burden for data collection. Much of the work described in this article focuses on hospitals and EMS, but patients are major players in outcomes as well. Delayed presentations confer poor outcomes, and a reliable way to capture ischemia duration would be helpful. In addition, future registries could include patient-reported outcomes for use as an effectiveness measure.

Rural populations face unresolved challenges in accessing emergency care for STEMI and other life-threatening conditions.[56,57] AMI mortality rates are higher and rising among critical access hospitals that treat rural populations compared with other hospitals.[58–60] Much of the work, described previously, excludes patients who transfer very late in the course of the disease or never make it to a PCI-capable hospital at all. Are dedicated registries needed for these non-transferred patients? Critical access and rural hospitals play a key role in triaging patients for rapid treatment and these hospitals are financially precarious in the United States health care system. Closures could affect both primary prevention efforts and triage and

transfer for STEMI care.[61] The COVID-19 pandemic has demonstrated the fragility of health care delivery systems. In the United States, during the course of the pandemic, the observed STEMI activation rate has declined, and the average D2B time at PCI-capable facilities has increased.[62,63] Importantly, the North American COVID-19 ST-Segment-Elevation Myocardial Infarction registry recently was announced to further investigate the STEMI population during the pandemic, which may reveal areas for improvement in these systems of care.[64]

Last, but certainly not least, vulnerable patient groups, such as women, racial/ethnic minorities, and the elderly, experience treatment

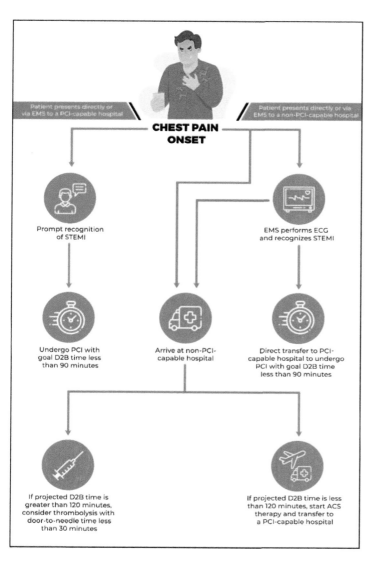

Fig. 1. Suggested treatment and transfer pathway for STEMI patients. A protocol to direct STEMI treatment in regional systems of care. ACS, acute coronary syndrome. (*Adapted from* O'Gara et al.[36])

delays. Some data suggest that regionalized, protocol-driven care has improved treatment and outcome disparities among vulnerable populations.[65,66] When minority and female patients were analyzed as a subset of the Mission: Lifeline Accelerator project, however, reperfusion times improved for male patients but not for minority and female patients.[67] As with almost every aspect of health care delivery in the United States, racism, sexism, and ageism must be actively combatted to improve outcomes for vulnerable populations with STEMI.

SUMMARY

Regional systems of care for STEMI have been developed successfully in the United States and beyond, with a positive impact on outcomes from this life-threatening condition. Key features of a successful STEMI regional system of care include

- Coordination between multiple stakeholders in STEMI care
- Ongoing data collection systems for rapid cycle learning
- Ability of EMS or ED physicians to activate the catheterization laboratory with a single call to a central dispatch
- Availability of a fully staffed catheterization laboratory within 30 minutes
- Regional protocols to allow for timely transfer of STEMI patients to PCI-capable hospitals, with a goal FMC-to-device time of less than or equal to 120 minutes for patients initially receiving care at a non–PCI-capable facility and less than or equal to 90 minutes for patients immediately brought to a PCI-capable facility
- Regular feedback to physicians, EMS personnel, and health system leadership

Based on the body of evidence supporting timely reperfusion in STEMI, the ACCF and the AHA released the 2013 guidelines for the management of STEMI, encouraging health systems to focus on time to reperfusion among eligible patients (Fig. 1; see Table 2). Similar recommendations are present in European Society of Cardiology (ESC) guidelines.[68] As presented in this article, the complex body of evidence for the optimization of STEMI care is ever-evolving. Thus, the national guidelines will continue to evolve, with a focus on improved patient care and decreased mortality and morbidity.

CLINICS CARE POINTS

- Successful outcomes for patients with ST elevation myocardial infarction starts with early recognition.
- Timely reperfusion leads to decreased morbidity and mortality.
- Patients presenting with cardiogenic shock and ST elevation myocardial infarction have high mortality rates, and transfer to a dedicated shock center should be considered.
- Implentation and maintenance of regional systems prevent delays in reperfusion time and improve patient outcomes.

DISCLOSURE

R.U. Shah reports grant support from the National Heart, Lung, and Blood Institute (NHLBI) (5K08HL136850) and additional research support from Women As One and the Doris Duke Foundation. All other authors have no disclosures to report.

REFERENCES

1. Keeley EC, Boura JA, Grines CL. Primary angioplasty versus intravenous thrombolytic therapy for acute myocardial infarction: a quantitative review of 23 randomised trials. Lancet 2003;361(9351): 13–20.
2. Van't Hof AWJ, Liem A, Suryapranata H. Clinical presentation and outcome of patients with early, intermediate and late reperfusion therapy by primary coronary angioplasty for acute myocardial infarction. Eur Heart J 1998. Available at: https://academic.oup.com/eurheartj/article-abstract/19/1/118/524518.
3. Alnasser SMA, Huang W, Gore JM, et al. Late consequences of acute coronary syndromes: Global registry of acute coronary events (GRACE) follow-up. Am J Med 2015;128(7):766–75.
4. Terkelsen CJ, Jensen LO, Tilsted H-H, et al. Health care system delay and heart failure in patients with st-segment elevation myocardial infarction treated with primary percutaneous coronary intervention: follow-up of population-based medical registry data. Ann Intern Med 2011;155(6):361.
5. Bradley Elizabeth H, Nallamothu Brahmajee K, Jeph H, et al. National Efforts to Improve Door-to-Balloon Time. J Am Coll Cardiol 2009;54(25): 2423–9.
6. Jollis JG, Al-Khalidi HR, Monk L, et al. Expansion of a Regional ST-segment–elevation myocardial infarction system to an entire state. Circulation 2012;126(2):189–95.
7. Eagle KA, Goodman SG, Avezum A, et al. Practice variation and missed opportunities for reperfusion

in ST-segment-elevation myocardial infarction: findings from the Global Registry of Acute Coronary Events (GRACE). Lancet 2002;359(9304):373–7.

8. Granger CB, Bates ER, Jollis JG, et al. Improving Care of STEMI in the United States 2008 to 2012. J Am Heart Assoc 2019;8(1):e008096.

9. McNamara RL, Wang Y, Herrin J, et al. Effect of door-to-balloon time on mortality in patients with ST-segment elevation myocardial infarction. J Am Coll Cardiol 2006;47(11):2180–6.

10. Masoudi FA, Ponirakis A, de Lemos JA, et al. Trends in U.S. Cardiovascular Care: 2016 Report From 4 ACC National Cardiovascular Data Registries. J Am Coll Cardiol 2017;69(11):1427–50.

11. Davies MJ, Woolf N, Robertson WB. Pathology of acute myocardial infarction with particular reference to occlusive coronary thrombi. Br Heart J 1976;38(7):659–64.

12. Grüntzig A. Transluminal dilatation of coronary-artery stenosis. Lancet 1978;311(8058):263.

13. Selection of reperfusion therapy for individual patients with evolving myocardial infarction. Eur Heart J 1997;18(9):1371–81.

14. Fischman DL, Leon MB, Baim DS, et al. A Randomized comparison of coronary-stent placement and balloon angioplasty in the treatment of coronary artery disease. N Engl J Med 1994; 331(8):496–501.

15. Widimský P, Budesínský T, Vorác D, et al. Long distance transport for primary angioplasty vs immediate thrombolysis in acute myocardial infarction. Final results of the randomized national multicentre trial–PRAGUE-2. Eur Heart J 2003;24(1):94–104.

16. Andersen HR, Nielsen TT, Rasmussen K, et al. A comparison of coronary angioplasty with fibrinolytic therapy in acute myocardial infarction. N Engl J Med 2003;349(8):733–42.

17. Henry TD, Sharkey SW, Nicholas Burke M, et al. A regional system to provide timely access to percutaneous coronary intervention for ST-elevation myocardial infarction. Circulation 2007; 116(7):721–8.

18. De Luca G, Harry S, Paul OJ, et al. Time delay to treatment and mortality in primary angioplasty for acute myocardial infarction. Circulation 2004; 109(10):1223–5.

19. Rathore SS, Curtis JP, Chen J, et al. Association of door-to-balloon time and mortality in patients admitted to hospital with ST elevation myocardial infarction: national cohort study. BMJ 2009;338:b1807.

20. Hani J, Daniel A, Bhatt Deepak L, et al. 2017 AHA/ACC clinical performance and quality measures for adults with ST-Elevation and non–ST-elevation myocardial infarction: a report of the American College of Cardiology/American Heart Association Task Force on Performance Measures. Circ Cardiovasc Qual Outcomes 2017;10(10):e000032.

21. Menees DS, Peterson ED, Wang Y, et al. Door-to-balloon time and mortality among patients undergoing primary PCI. N Engl J Med 2013;369(10): 901–9.

22. Nallamothu BK, Normand S-LT, Wang Y, et al. Relation between door-to-balloon times and mortality after primary percutaneous coronary intervention over time: a retrospective study. Lancet 2015; 385(9973):1114–22.

23. Dauerman Harold L, Bates Eric R, Kontos Michael C, et al. Nationwide analysis of patients with st-segment–elevation myocardial infarction transferred for primary percutaneous intervention. Circ Cardiovasc Interv 2015;8(5):e002450.

24. Wang TY, Nallamothu BK, Krumholz HM, et al. Association of door-in to door-out time with reperfusion delays and outcomes among patients transferred for primary percutaneous coronary intervention. JAMA 2011;305(24):2540–7.

25. Jollis JG, Al-Khalidi HR, Roettig ML, et al. Regional systems of care demonstration project: american heart association mission: lifeline STEMI systems accelerator. Circulation 2016;134(5):365–74.

26. O'Gara Patrick T, Kushner Frederick G, Ascheim Deborah D, et al. 2013 ACCF/AHA guideline for the management of ST-elevation myocardial infarction. Circulation 2013;127(4):e362–425.

27. Rokos IC, French WJ, Koenig WJ, et al. Integration of pre-hospital electrocardiograms and ST-elevation myocardial infarction receiving center (SRC) networks: impact on door-to-balloon times across 10 independent regions. JACC Cardiovasc Interv 2009;2(4):339–46.

28. Scholz KH, Friede T, Meyer T, et al. Prognostic significance of emergency department bypass in stable and unstable patients with ST-segment elevation myocardial infarction. Eur Heart J Acute Cardiovasc Care 2020;9(1_suppl):34–44.

29. Ting HH, Krumholz HM, Bradley EH, et al. Implementation and integration of prehospital ECGs into systems of care for acute coronary syndrome: a scientific statement from the American Heart Association Interdisciplinary Council on Quality of Care and Outcomes Research, Emergency Cardiovascular Care Committee, Council on Cardiovascular Nursing, and Council on Clinical Cardiology. Circulation 2008;118(10):1066–79.

30. Stowens JC, Sonnad SS, Rosenbaum RA. Using EMS dispatch to trigger STEMI alerts decreases door-to-balloon times. West J Emerg Med 2015; 16(3):472–80.

31. Kobayashi A, Misumida N, Aoi S, et al. STEMI notification by EMS predicts shorter door-to-balloon time and smaller infarct size. Am J Emerg Med 2016;34(8):1610–3.

32. Langabeer JR, Henry TD, Kereiakes DJ, et al. Growth in percutaneous coronary intervention on

capacity relative to population and disease prevalence. J Am Heart Assoc 2013;2(6):e000370.

33. McNamara RL, Herrin J, Wang Y, et al. Impact of delay in door-to-needle time on mortality in patients with ST-segment elevation myocardial infarction. Am J Cardiol 2007;100(8):1227–32.

34. Newby LK, Rutsch WR, Califf RM, et al. Time from symptom onset to treatment and outcomes after thrombolytic therapy. GUSTO-1 Investigators. J Am Coll Cardiol 1996;27(7):1645–55.

35. Boersma E, Maas AC, Deckers JW, et al. Early thrombolytic treatment in acute myocardial infarction: reappraisal of the golden hour. Lancet 1996; 348(9030):771–5.

36. O'Gara PT, Kushner FG, Ascheim DD, et al. 2013 ACCF/AHA guidelines for the management of ST-elevation myocaridal infarction: executive summary. Circulation 2013;127(4):529–55.

37. Jollis JG, Roettig ML, Aluko AO, et al. Implementation of a statewide system for coronary reperfusion for ST-segment elevation myocardial infarction. JAMA 2007;298(20):2371–80.

38. DelliFraine J, Langabeer J 2nd, Segrest W, et al. Developing an ST-elevation myocardial infarction system of care in Dallas County. Am Heart J 2013; 165(6):926–31.

39. Rokos IC, Larson DM, Henry TD, et al. Rationale for establishing regional ST-elevation myocardial infarction receiving center (SRC) networks. Am Heart J 2006;152(4):661–7.

40. Puymirat E, Simon T, Cayla G, et al. Acute myocardial infarction: changes in patient characteristics, management, and 6-month outcomes over a period of 20 years in the FAST-MI Program (French Registry of Acute ST-Elevation or Non-ST-Elevation Myocardial Infarction) 1995 to 2015. Circulation 2017;136(20):1908–19.

41. Kalla K, Christ G, Karnik R, et al. Implementation of Guidelines Improves the Standard of Care. Circulation 2006;113(20):2398–405.

42. Park J, Choi KH, Lee JM, et al. Prognostic implications of door-to-balloon time and onset-to-door time on mortality in patients with ST-segment–elevation myocardial infarction treated with primary percutaneous coronary intervention. J Am Heart Assoc 2019;8(9):e012188.

43. Chan AW, Kornder J, Elliott H, et al. Improved survival associated with pre-hospital triage strategy in a large regional ST-segment elevation myocardial infarction program. JACC Cardiovasc Interv 2012; 5(12):1239–46.

44. Yeh RW, Sidney S, Chandra M, et al. Population trends in the incidence and outcomes of acute myocardial infarction. N Engl J Med 2010;362(23): 2155–65.

45. Shah RU, Henry TD, Rutten-Ramos S, et al. Increasing percutaneous coronary interventions for ST-segment elevation myocardial infarction in the United States: progress and opportunity. JACC Cardiovasc Interv 2015;8(1 Pt B):139–46.

46. Granger CB, Bates ER, Jollis JG, et al. Improving care of STEMI in the United States 2008 to 2012: a report from the American Heart Association Mission: lifeline program. J Am Heart Assoc 2019; 8(1):e008096.

47. Farshid A, Allada C, Chandrasekhar J, et al. Shorter ischaemic time and improved survival with pre-hospital STEMI diagnosis and direct transfer for primary PCI. Heart Lung Circ 2015;24(3):234–40.

48. Scholz KH, Maier SKG, Maier LS, et al. Impact of treatment delay on mortality in ST-segment elevation myocardial infarction (STEMI) patients presenting with and without haemodynamic instability: results from the German prospective, multicentre FITT-STEMI trial. Eur Heart J 2018;39(13):1065–74.

49. Benjamin EJ, Blaha MJ, Chiuve SE, et al. Heart disease and stroke statistics—2017 update: a report from the American Heart Association. Circulation 2017;135:e146.

50. Miller L. Cardiogenic shock in acute myocardial infarction: the era of mechanical support. J Am Coll Cardiol 2016;67:1881.

51. Rab T, Ratanapo S, Kern K, et al. Cardiac Shock Care Centers. J Am Coll Cardiol 2018;72(16): 1972–80.

52. Vallabhajosyla S, Prasad A, Bell M, et al. Extracorporeal membrane oxygenation use in acute myocardial infarction in the United States, 2000 to 2014. Circ Heart Fail 2019;12:e005929.

53. Taleb I, Koliopoulou AG, Tandar A, et al. Shock team approach to refractory cardiogenic shock requiring short term mechanical circulatory support: a proof of concept. Circulation 2019;140:98–100.

54. Tehrani B, Truesdell A, Singh R, et al. Implementation of a cardiogenic shock team and clinical outcomes (INOVA-SHOCK Registry_: Observation and retrospective study. JMIR Res Protoc 2018; 7(6):e160.

55. Muntner P, Hardy ST, Fine LJ, et al. Trends in Blood pressure control among US adults with hypertension, 1999-2000 to 2017-2018. JAMA 2020. https:// doi.org/10.1001/jama.2020.14545.

56. Johnston KJ, Wen H, Joynt Maddox KE. Lack of access to specialists associated with mortality and preventable hospitalizations of rural medicare beneficiaries. Health Aff 2019;38(12):1993–2002.

57. Harrington RA, Califf RM, Balamurugan A, et al. Call to action: rural health: a presidential advisory from the American Heart Association and American Stroke Association. Circulation 2020;141(10):e615–44.

58. Joynt KE, John Orav E, Jha AK. Mortality rates for medicare beneficiaries admitted to critical access and non–critical access hospitals, 2002-2010. JAMA 2013;309(13):1379–87.

59. Bhuyan SS, Wang Y, Opoku S, et al. Rural-urban differences in acute myocardial infarction mortality: evidence from Nebraska. J Cardiovasc Dis Res 2013;4(4):209–13.

60. Bechtold D, Salvatierra GG, Bulley E, et al. Geographic variation in treatment and outcomes among patients with AMI: investigating urban-rural differences among hospitalized patients. J Rural Health 2017;33(2):158–66.

61. Bai G, Yehia F, Chen W, et al. Varying trends in the financial viability of US Rural Hospitals, 2011-17. Health Aff 2020;39(6):942–8.

62. Garcia S, Albaghdadi MS, Meraj PM, et al. Reduction in ST-segment elevation cardiac catheterization laboratory activations in the united states during COVID-19 Pandemic. J Am Coll Cardiol 2020;75(22):2871–2.

63. Gluckman TJ, Wilson MA, Chiu S-T, et al. Case rates, treatment approaches, and outcomes in acute myocardial infarction during the coronavirus disease 2019 pandemic. JAMA Cardiol 2020. https://doi.org/10.1001/jamacardio.2020.3629.

64. Dehghani P, Davidson LJ, Grines CL, et al. North American COVID-19 ST-Segment-Elevation Myocardial Infarction (NACMI) registry: rationale, design, and implications. Am Heart J 2020;227:11–8.

65. Glickman SW, Granger CB, Ou F-S, et al. Impact of a statewide ST-segment–elevation myocardial infarction regionalization program on treatment times for women, minorities, and the elderly. Circ Cardiovasc Qual Outcomes 2010;3(5):514–21.

66. Edmund Anstey D, Li S, Thomas L, et al. Race and sex differences in management and outcomes of patients after ST-Elevation and Non-ST-elevation myocardial infarct: results from the NCDR. Clin Cardiol 2016;39(10):585–95.

67. Hinohara TT, Al-Khalidi HR, Fordyce CB, et al. Impact of regional systems of care on disparities in care among female and black patients presenting with ST-segment–elevation myocardial infarction. J Am Heart Assoc 2017;6(10):e007122.

68. Ibanez B, James S, Agewall S, Antunes MJ. 2017 ESC Guidelines for the management of acute myocardial infarction in patients presenting with ST-segment elevation: The Task Force for the management of …. Eur Heart J 2018;.https://academic.oup.com/eurheartj/article-abstract/39/2/119/4095042.

Prehospital Evaluation, ED Management, Transfers, and Management of Inpatient STEMI

Alayn Govea, MD[a,b], Jerry Lipinksi, MD[b,c],
Mitul P. Patel, MD, FSCAI[b,d],*

KEYWORDS

- ST elevation myocardial infarction • STEMI management • STEMI transfers
- Emergency department STEMI care • Myocardial infarction • Inpatient STEMI
- ST elevation differential diagnosis

KEY POINTS

- High index of suspicion and prompt diagnosis with electrocardiogram (ECG) within 10 minutes of medical contact reduce first medical contact to revascularization time and mortality.
- Percutaneous coronary intervention (PCI) is preferred over thrombolytics, and prehospital activation of a cardiac catheterization team reduces time to reperfusion. Transfers requiring greater than or equal to 120 minutes should receive fibrinolytics.
- Emergency departments must stabilize unstable patients and evaluate for other life-threatening conditions or contraindications to coronary intervention.
- Full-dose aspirin; anticoagulation with heparin, enoxaparin, or bivalirudin; and P2Y12 inhibition with ticagrelor, prasugrel, clopidogrel (less preferred), or intravenous cangrelor are recommended for ST elevation myocardial infarction (STEMI) patients.
- In-hospital STEMI patients may show atypical symptoms or are unable to express themselves; therefore, changes in clinical status or telemetry could warrant further evaluation.

INTRODUCTION AND DEFINITIONS

ST elevation myocardial infarction (STEMI) is a clinical syndrome composed of symptoms of myocardial infarction in association with ST-segment elevation on electrocardiography (ECG) followed by release of biomarkers of myocardial necrosis. Between 2008 and 2011, the prevalence of STEMI decreased from 133 to 55 cases per 100,000 person-years and represents between 25% and 40% of acute myocardial infarctions.[1] Between 2001 and 2011, in-hospital mortality for patients with STEMI who received either coronary artery bypass grafting or percutaneous coronary intervention (PCI) remained unchanged, but mortality was substantially higher and increased for those not undergoing revascularization (12.43% to 14.91%).[1] Societal guidelines have focused on early identification and revascularization to improve cardiovascular outcomes; as a result, STEMIs leading to heart failure have decreased from 46% to 28% in a Swedish registry study of 199,851 patients.[2] This review covers the general management strategies and identifies key guidelines for patients with STEMI in the prehospital, emergency

[a] Division of Cardiovascular Medicine, UC San Diego, San Diego, CA, USA; [b] UC San Diego Sulpizio Cardiovascular Center, 9452 Medical Center Drive #7411, La Jolla, CA 92037, USA; [c] Department of Internal Medicine, UC San Diego, San Diego, CA, USA; [d] Division of Cardiovascular Medicine, UC San Diego Cardiovascular Institute, San Diego, CA, USA
* Corresponding author.
E-mail address: mpatel@health.ucsd.edu

Intervent Cardiol Clin 10 (2021) 293–306
https://doi.org/10.1016/j.iccl.2021.03.002

department (ED), and in-hospital settings and examines key aspects of care for interhospital transfer patients.

Initial identification of STEMI remains one of the most important facets of care. ECG is critical for diagnosis of STEMI, and myocardial infarction markers may not be elevated in the early presentation of myocardial infarction. The European Society of Cardiology (ESC)/American College of Cardiology Foundation (ACCF)/ American Heart Association (AHA)/World Heart Federation Task Force for the Universal Definition of Myocardial Infarction classifies diagnostic ST elevations (STEs) as new J-point elevations, in the absence of left bundle branch block (LBBB) and left ventricular hypertrophy (LVH), of greater than or equal to 1 mm in at least 2 contiguous leads except V2-V3. V2-V3 require greater than or equal to 2.5-mm elevation in men less than 40 years old, greater than or equal to 2-mm elevation in men over 40 years old, or greater than or equal to 1.5-mm elevation in women.[3,4] Evolving STEMIs develop new pathologic Q waves in the transmural infarct territory. ST depressions represent reciprocal changes and may accompany STEMIs although not always may be present. New LBBB has been considered STEMI equivalent; however, upon initial presentation, its acuity often is unclear. In isolation, LBBB without other clinical symptoms of myocardial infarction should not be considered diagnostic of acute coronary syndrome (ACS).[3,5]

Standard 12-lead ECGs may not always yield clear STEs in patients presenting with symptoms of transmural myocardial injury, and supplemental ECGs must be obtained to confirm a STEMI diagnosis. Patients may present very early before the development of STE. In this scenario, ECG may show hyperacute T waves, and repeat ECGs should be performed in short intervals to assess for evolving STEs. Electrographically silent myocardial infarctions may occur with left circumflex coronary artery occlusions or occlusions of bypass grafts. These infarcts should be suspected in patients presenting with signs of a myocardial infarction without clear ECG changes and should prompt a posterior ECG with leads V7-V9, which can identify STEMI in many of these patients (Fig. 1).[3,5,6] Inferobasal STEMIs (previously known as posterior infarcts) may present with isolated ST depressions of greater than or equal to 0.5-mm in leads V1-V3, especially when the terminal T wave is positive. If these are present, a posterior ECG showing STE greater than or equal to 0.5 mm in V7-V9 (≥1 mm in men <40 years old) can confirm the diagnosis. Elevations in aVR greater

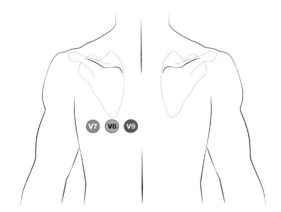

Fig. 1. Posterior ECG lead placement. (*From* Cadogan M. Posterior Myocardial Infarction • LITFL. Published 2019. Accessed October 30, 2020. https://litfl.com/posterior-myocardial-infarction-ecg-library/.)

than or equal to 1-mm STE with diffuse ST depression in greater than or equal to 8 leads suggest multivessel ischemia or left main coronary obstruction, particularly if hemodynamic instability is present.[4,5] Lastly, in patients with inferior infarcts, leads V1 or aVR may exhibit STE greater than or equal to 1 mm, and obtaining a right-sided ECG with leads V3R and V4R is indicated (Fig. 2).[7] ST elevation greater than or equal to 0.5 mm (≥1 mm in men <30 years old) suggests right ventricular (RV) infarct.[4]

Clinical Care Points: Introduction and Definition

- Diagnostic STEs are new J-point elevations, in the absence of LBBB and

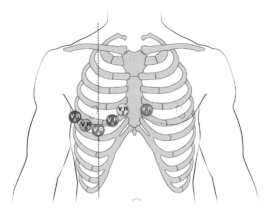

Fig. 2. Right-sided ECG lead placement. (*From* Cadogan M. Posterior Myocardial Infarction • LITFL. Published 2019. Accessed October 30, 2020. https://litfl.com/posterior-myocardial-infarction-ecg-library/.)

LVH, of greater than or equal to 1 mm in at least 2 contiguous leads except V2-V3. V2-V3 require greater than or equal to 2.5-mm elevation in men less than 40 years old, greater than or equal to 2-mm elevation in men over 40 years old, or greater than or equal to 1.5-mm elevation in women[3,4]

- Electrographically silent myocardial infarctions or inferobasal STEMIs may require a posterior ECG for diagnosis (V7-V9)
- For patients with inferior STE, a right-sided ECG is indicated to diagnose RV involvement

PREHOSPITAL EVALUATION

Emergency medical services (EMS) provide an essential role in the STEMI response system because they serve as the first medical contact (FMC) for patients activating 9-1-1 for symptoms of chest pain. Their initial evaluation must focus on rapid assessment of vitals, stability, symptoms, and obtaining an initial ECG.

In 2007, the AHA introduced the Mission: Lifeline program, which established systems of care for STEMI patients aimed at improving the quality of care in STEMI patients.[8] As part of these, FMC-to-device (FMC2D) time became a key metric. It includes the prehospital period and door-to-balloon time (DTBT), reflecting the efficiency of the totality of STEMI care. To reduce FMC2D time, the AHA emphasized prehospital ECGs, paramedic consultation with ED physician and/or cardiologist, and prehospital activation of a cardiac catheterization laboratory (CCL) STEMI team.

EMS personnel must have a high suspicion for STEMI, especially in patients with risk factors, such as diabetes, tobacco use, end-stage renal disease, hyperlipidemia, and hypertension. In all patients with chest pain, an ECG should be obtained as soon as possible after stabilization of the patient. Women and diabetics may have atypical symptoms, such as heartburn or epigastric pain, and paramedics should have a low threshold to obtain an ECG. Prior to the introduction of the AHA Mission: Lifeline program, fewer than 10% of STEMI patients received a prehospital ECG despite evidence demonstrating a reduction in DTBT and FMC2D time.[9–11] Wide adoption of prehospital ECG has encountered several barriers, including funding for ECG and transmission equipment and paramedic training for accurate ECG interpretation.[12]

The AHA recommends interpretation of ECG by paramedics, the ECG computer algorithm, and ECG transmission for remote assessment by a physician. Use of these resources depends on local protocol, availability of funding, and system-wide implementation of best practices. Paramedics can be trained to interpret ECGs and, in combination with a computer-based algorithm, their sensitivity can vary between 71% and 97%, with specificity ranging from 91% to 100%.[9] This strategy can lead to higher false-positive rates and false negative rates, however, when compared with physician interpretation.[9] Ideally, paramedics would transmit the ECG to an on-call cardiologist or ED physician for confirmation and management decisions; however, the availability of this technology may be limited, especially in rural areas (limited wireless coverage) or in a moving ambulance (limited or absent cellular signal), resulting in failed transmission or delays in up to 20% to 44% of cases.[9] Transmission of the ECG to the ED or cardiology provider not only decreases false CCL activations but also allows for early activation of the CCL staff, resulting in greater likelihood of reaching the laboratory with FMC2D time less than or equal to 90 minutes (76.6% vs 68.6%, respectively), shorter door-to-device time (40 min [interquartile ratio (IQR): 30–51 min] vs 52 min [IQR: 41–65 min], respectively), and lower in-hospital mortality (2.8% vs 3.4%, respectively; $P = .01$).[13]

In January 2020, the AHA Mission: Lifeline program released additional guidelines outlining criteria for prehospital activation and direct to CCL criteria aimed at reducing time to reperfusion (Fig. 3).[12] Prehospital activation should occur in 2 scenarios:

1. If the ED physician or cardiologist on call receives the prehospital ECG and determines that it meets STEMI criteria
2. If transmission is not available, then the EMS should notify the ED of STEMI if the ECG shows greater than 1-mm STE in 2 or more contiguous leads or if the machine interprets STEMI.

To shorten reperfusion time further, the AHA proposed direct to CCL criteria aimed at identifying patients who are hemodynamically stable, with a clear STEMI, and who have no contraindications or other conditions requiring triage by the emergency room staff (see Fig. 3) and who can be taken directly from the ambulance to the CCL. This strategy has been poorly adopted due to concerns over false CCL activations, the

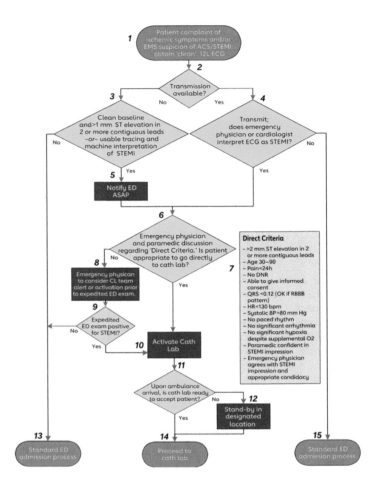

Fig. 3. Prehospital STEMI management algorithm (PreACT) recommended by the AHA/ACC. (*From* Kontos MC, Gunderson MR, Zegre-Hemsey JK, et al. Prehospital Activation of Hospital Resources (PREACT) ST-Segment–Elevation Myocardial Infarction (STEMI): A Standardized Approach to Prehospital Activation and Direct to the Catheterization Laboratory for STEMI Recommendations *From* the American Heart Association's Mission: Lifeline Program. J Am Heart Assoc. 2020,9(2). https://doi.org/10.1161/JAHA.119.011963.)

need to monitor patients until the CCL team arrives, lack of consensus on direct to CCL criteria, and limited resources during off-duty hours.[12]

Upon confirmation of STEMI, the patient should be transported, preferably to a nearby, PCI-capable hospital rather than the closest ED.[3] Paramedics should place patients on continuous telemetry and monitor for arrhythmias, hemodynamic instability, or signs of cardiogenic shock, such as tachycardia, hypotension, cool extremities, and altered mental status. Patients should receive an oral dose of plain aspirin (non–enteric-coated formulation), 162 mg to 325 mg, in accordance with AHA guidelines.[3] If the oral route is not feasible, rectal aspirin should be administered.

Relief of chest pain confers a reduction in sympathetic activation, decreasing vasoconstriction and reducing the workload of the myocardium. Sublingual nitroglycerin can be used to relieve ischemic symptoms and longer-acting nitroglycerin ointments could be used, if available. Caution must be taken when using nitroglycerin in patients with STEs in the inferior leads because some of these patients may be experiencing a concomitant RV infarct, in which case nitroglycerin can result in severe hypotension and shock. Historically, intravenous (IV) narcotics have been used in this setting; however, recent series have suggested that morphine administration can reduce antiplatelet drug absorption and its active metabolite level.[14] STEMI patients who received morphine prior to P2Y12 inhibitors demonstrated higher platelet reactivity and reduced endogenous thrombolysis within the first 24 hours of antiplatelet therapy administration.[15,16] Morphine use prior to PCI is independently associated with larger infarct size and lower myocardial salvage index on magnetic resonance imaging (MRI).[17] Despite increased myocardial injury, retrospective analysis of the Does Cyclosporine Improve Outcome in ST Elevation Myocardial Infarction Patients (CIRCUS) did not show an increase in all-cause death, cardiovascular death, heart failure, cardiogenic shock, recurrent myocardial infarction, unstable angina, and stroke at 1 year in 969 patients.[18] Oxygen therapy is indicated in hypoxic patients with an arterial oxygen saturation less than 90%. In patients with normal oxygen saturations, routine administration of oxygen does not improve symptoms or reduce infarct size but may result in harm, as evidenced by higher creatinine kinase and larger infarct size on cardiac MRI at 6 months.[19] Thus, routine use of oxygen in patients with saturations greater than 90% is not recommended.[3]

Primary PCI is the preferred reperfusion strategy in STEMI patients within 12 hours of symptom onset in those who can be transported to an appropriately equipped and staffed, high-volume center within 120 minutes from STEMI diagnosis.[3] If a delay of greater than 120 minutes is anticipated, fibrinolytic therapy is indicated.

In the United States, prehospital fibrinolytics have yet to receive a recommendation in the guidelines and are not used. Rural areas often lack the resources for proper training of paramedics and funding for the necessary equipment. Administration of fibrinolytics in the prehospital setting reduced FMC to thrombolysis time by at least 38 minutes in 2 meta-analyses, encompassing 7 trials.[20-22] Clinical outcomes data supporting prehospital administration of fibrinolytics are heterogenic and strong evidence is lacking. A meta-analysis of 6 trials with 6434 patients showed a decrease in mortality (odds ratio 0.83; 95% CI, 0.70–0.98) in patients treated with prehospital fibrinolytics versus in-hospital fibrinolytics. A subsequent Cochrane review of 3 randomized trials concluded with low-quality evidence that there was no difference in mortality between the 2 groups. Both of these meta-analyses only included trials with patients undergoing a fibrinolytic strategy and PCI patients were not included. The CAPTIM study demonstrated a reduction in 5-year mortality in patients who received prehospital fibrinolytics (time to treatment 130 minutes) within 2 hours of the onset of symptoms and then transferred to PCI-capable center compared with PCI strategy alone (time to treatment, 190 minutes), hazard ratio 0.5% (95% CI, 0.25–0.98). After 2 hours of symptoms there was no difference in mortality.[23] The STREAM trial, published in 2013, randomized patients presenting within 3 hours of symptom onset and who were unable to undergo PCI within 1 hour to either fibrinolytic therapy followed by PCI versus PCI alone. Although the fibrinolytic group showed improved Thrombolysis in Myocardial Infarction (TIMI) flow at initial angiography, the groups did not differ in the primary composite endpoint of death from any cause, shock, congestive heart failure, or reinfarction up to 30 days, even in those patients randomized to fibrinolytics within 2 hours of symptoms onset. Patients receiving fibrinolytics had slightly increased rise of intracranial hemorrhages (1.0% vs 0.2%, respectively; P = .04); although, after implementing the reduced dose of tenecteplase for patients greater than or equal to 75 years old, the statistical difference was abolished (0.5% vs 0.3%, respectively; P = .45).[24]

Clinical Care Points: Prehospital Evaluation

- As part of the prehospital evaluation the AHA recommends a prehospital ECG, paramedic consultation with physician and transmission of ECG, and prehospital activation of CCL STEMI team.
- FMC2D time is a key metric evaluating the efficiency of hospital and county-wide systems of care when treating STEMI patients.
- Upon confirmation of STEMI, the patient should be transported preferably to the closest PCI-capable hospital rather than the closest ED.
- Full-dose aspirin may be administered by EMS personnel en route to hospital. Sublingual nitroglycerine also may be given to relieve chest pain but must be used with caution in patients with inferior infarcts due to possible RV involvement.
- Morphine and oxygen should not be administered routinely. Oxygen is indicated in patients with oxygen saturation of less than or equal to 90%.
- When using fibrinolytics as a reperfusion strategy, prehospital fibrinolytics are used in Europe but not in the United States because clinical outcomes data are heterogenic and strong evidence is lacking.

EMERGENCY DEPARTMENT MANAGEMENT

The ED's primary role is to confirm the STEMI diagnosis in patients arriving via ambulance, stabilize the patient, conduct further assessment to rule out alternative diagnostic possibilities or potential complications of myocardial infraction, and assess for any contraindications to proceeding to a CCL. Patients with chest pain who do not arrive by ambulance must be triaged and an ECG must be performed within 10 minutes of arrival to the ED. Upon detection of STEMI, the patient should be given a full-dose aspirin and be assessed immediately by an ED physician.

For all patients arriving to the ED, either direct or by ambulance, the ED physician should consult with the on-call cardiology team. Telemetry monitoring and assessment of the patient's hemodynamic stability and respiratory status should be performed concurrently. For patients whose ECG was performed in the ambulance, a confirmatory ECG may be needed in the ED. After a diagnosis of STEMI is confirmed, activation of the CCL must occur expeditiously. Depending on the hospital protocol and staffing, ED physicians may be able to activate the CCL directly or may require activation by the on-call cardiologist. The 2013 AHA/ACC STEMI guidelines recommend protocols allowing ED or EMS personnel to activate the CCL, which may result in up to 65% false activations.[25] Implementation of the AHA Mission: Lifeline Pre-Act STEMI algorithm reduced false CCL from 54% to 14% to 15% in 1 series and resulted in earlier intervention for a majority of STEMI patients. After stabilization, limited history and physical examination focusing on ruling in or ruling out conditions that may mimic STE or that prohibit a patient from going to the CCL should be performed. Box 1 provides a review of the differential diagnosis for STEs on ECG.[26] Although this work-up is important for proper triaging and screening of patients prior to transport to CCL, it typically is performed after activation of the CCL to avoid delays in transporting the patient to the CCL.

There remains a population of patients in whom a delay in CCL transport from the ED is appropriate. Hemodynamically unstable patients or those in respiratory distress should be stabilized with the required vasopressor support, antiarrhythmic, or airway protection prior to transport to the CCL. Additionally, relative contraindications to anticoagulation should be reviewed and, for patients who may have suffered trauma, appropriate imaging is needed to limit the risk of a catastrophic bleed. Patients considered for additional work-up include trauma patients, those with unwitnessed cardiac arrest with unknown head trauma or neurologic deficits, and those found unconscious. Aortic dissections can cause severe chest pain and a may cause STEMI on ECG when there is involvement of the ascending aorta and coronary

Box 1
Differential diagnosis for ST elevations on electrocardiogram
Acute myocardial infarction
Prinzmetal angina
Early repolarization
LVH
LBBB
Acute pericarditis
Myocarditis
Ventricular aneurysm
Post-DC cardioversion
Myocardial tumor
Myocardial trauma
Brugada-type patterns
Massive pulmonary embolism
Hyperkalemia
Hypercalcemia
Hypothermia
Neurologic stress cardiomyopathy
Data from Wang K, Asinger RW, Marriott HJL. ST-Segment Elevation in Conditions Other Than Acute Myocardial Infarction. N Engl J Med. 2003; 349(22):2128-2135. https://doi.org/10.1056/nejmra 022580.

arteries. This subgroup of patients requires emergency surgery, with mortality increasing by 1% to 2% each hour after onset of symptoms; therefore, a high index of suspicion and rapid diagnosis is essential.[27] Lastly the wishes and desire of the patient or surrogate decision maker should be considered. Some considerations that require further discussion include elderly patients who wish to avoid resuscitation and do not wish to undergo procedures.

While waiting for transport to the CCL, AHA/ACC guidelines recommend administration of full-dose aspirin if not performed by EMS personnel and initiation of anticoagulation with unfractionated heparin (UFH), enoxaparin, or bivalirudin. Data from the per protocol analysis of the ATOLL trial suggest enoxaparin was superior to UFH in reducing the composite endpoint of 30-day death, myocardial infraction, procedural failure, or major bleeding in patients with STEMI undergoing primary PCI; however, the trial did not meet the primary endpoint in the intention-to-treat analysis.[28] Subsequently, a meta-analysis of 23 trials representing 30,966 patients, of whom 10,243 underwent primary PCI, showed a reduction in death, complications of myocardial infraction, and major bleeding events with the use of enoxaparin compared with heparin.[29] The AHA/ACC 2013 STEMI guidelines recommend the use of UFH for the management of STEMI patients but the more recent 2017 ESC guidelines state that enoxaparin should be considered in this setting.[3,5]

Dual antiplatelet therapy for 1 year is indicated in all patients with STEMI, according to the AHA/ACC guidelines. For patients undergoing primary PCI, the primary purpose of P2Y12 inhibition is to prevent stent thrombosis, but the optimal timing of P2Y12 therapy is less clear. Pharmacokinetic data suggest that early administration of P2Y12 inhibitors allows for optimal platelet inhibition prior to placement of stent. Observational data and a small trial of 300 patients suggest that administration of clopidogrel in the prehospital setting reduced post-PCI in-hospital mortality, reinfarction, and urgent target vessel revascularization[30,31]; however, both ESC and AHA/ACC guidelines recommend ticagrelor or prasugrel over clopidogrel in ACS because both have a faster onset of action, typically within 1 hour of administration.[32,33] Prasugrel carries a boxed warning in the United States for patients with a history of transient ischemic attack/stroke as well as those aged greater than or equal to 75 years because there is an increased risk of fatal and intracranial bleeding.[34] The Administration of Ticagrelor in the Cath Lab or in the Ambulance for New ST Elevation Myocardial Infarction to Open the Coronary Artery (ATLANTIC) trial assessed ticagrelor administration in the prehospital setting compared with in-hospital administration. The primary outcomes were resolution of STE of at least 70% prior to PCI and the proportion of patients who had TIMI 2 or better flow prior to PCI. These endpoints were not met. Despite pharmacokinetic data on 37 patients, suggesting no difference in platelet reactivity at any of the prespecified time points between the 2 groups, the rates of definite stent thrombosis were lower at 24 hours and at 30 days in those patients pretreated with ticagrelor (0% vs 0.8%, respectively, in the first 24 hours; 0.2% vs 1.2%, respectively, at 30 days).[35]

The parenteral P2Y12 inhibitor cangrelor and glycoprotein IIb/IIIa inhibitors, such as tirofiban, eptifibatide, and abciximab, are used more frequently in settings where administration of oral P2Y12 inhibitors is challenging, such as in cardiogenic shock with concomitant respiratory failure or when there may be a need for emergency surgery. The CANTIC study assessed cangrelor bolus and infusion with oral ticagrelor loading and showed that platelet inhibition occurs within 5 minutes of cangrelor administration and persisted through the infusion period.[36] More recently, the FABOLUS-FASTER trial showed tirofiban had superior platelet inhibition compared with both cangrelor and oral load of prasugrel alone.[37] This trial was limited to pharmacodynamic data and no clinical information on bleeding risk or stent thrombosis was reported.

In patients receiving fibrinolytics, an oral loading dose of clopidogrel, 300 mg, is recommended for those less than 75 years old, followed by 75 mg daily for 1 year. For patients greater than or equal to 75 years old, a loading dose is not recommended, and patients should be given a daily, 75-mg, dose.[3] Ticagrelor has been shown to have comparable TIMI major bleeding risk (1%–2%) and efficacy endpoints (death from vascular causes, myocardial infarction, stroke, severe recurrent ischemia, transient ischemic attack, or other arterial thrombotic events) compared with clopidogrel in STEMI patients treated with fibrinolytics.[38,39] Prasugrel has not been studied in this setting and neither ticagrelor nor prasugrel is recommended after fibrinolytics in the 2013 AHA/ACC STEMI guidelines.[3]

With the lack of strong evidence and physiologic plausibility, it is reasonable to recommend early administration of P2Y12 inhibitors, preferably ticagrelor or prasugrel, prior to transport to a catheterization laboratory. If a patient is transferred to the catheterization laboratory prior to P2Y12 administration, then a parenteral P2Y12 inhibitor or glycoprotein IIb/IIIa inhibitor should be considered, followed by a loading dose of the desired oral P2Y12 inhibitor. Currently, there is insufficient clinical evidence to recommend the use of parenteral P2Y12 inhibitors or IIb/IIIa inhibitors routinely, but their rapid onset and potency make them well suited for use in specific clinical scenarios.

Particular caution must be taken when RV infarct is suspected. Providers should have a high suspicion for RV infarcts in inferior STEMI. In this setting, obtaining a right-sided ECG can prove invaluable. Nitrates in this setting are contraindicated because they reduce preload in a highly preload-dependent situation, especially in the setting of RV dysfunction from an acute myocardial infarction. IV volume expansion is most important in the management of hypotension in these patients. Additionally, electrical disturbances, such as complete heart block or sinus node dysfunction, may occur, resulting in bradyarrhythmias. Managing teams must be prepared to transcutaneous pace these patients and, if required, place a temporary transvenous pacemaker.

Clinical Care Points: Emergency Department Management

- The ED's primary role is confirmation of STEMIs arriving by ambulance, triaging self-presenting patients with ECG within 10 minutes of arrival, stabilization of unstable patients, and assessing for alternative diagnosis and for contraindications to PCI. This should be performed in consultation with the on-call cardiology team to prevent delays in care.
- Guidelines recommend administration of full-dose aspirin; anticoagulation with heparin, enoxaparin, or bivalirudin; and P2Y12 inhibition, preferably with ticagrelor or prasugrel.
- Sublingual, IV, or transdermal nitrates can be used for chest pain relief, although caution must be taken if RV infarct is suspected. IV morphine should be used cautiously.

MANAGEMENT OF TRANSFER ST ELEVATION MYOCARDIAL INFARCTION PATIENTS

In recent years, there has been an expansion of freestanding EDs in suburban and rural locations across the United States. Although the expansion has increased access to care, there is the unfortunate downside of patients presenting to these facilities with STEMI for which they cannot offer immediate access to primary PCI; as such, these freestanding EDs and small hospitals tend to have transfer agreements in place for patients presenting with acute STEMI. This puts an incredible onus on the EDs as well as physicians from smaller hospitals to be in direct contact with a PCI-capable institution such that a patient can be transferred for primary PCI. Furthermore, logistics play an important role in determining whether a patient should be treated with a facilitated PCI strategy or managed with a pharmacoinvasive approach while transferring to a higher level of care. In some situations, appropriate ground or air transport can be arranged in time for facilitated PCI but limited resources restrict their use. According to the 2013 ACCF/AHA guidelines, if a patient were to present with STEMI at a non–PCI-capable facility and the treating team can achieve DTBT of less than 120 minutes, including transfer time, then primary PCI should be attempted.[3] Implementation of strategies to reduce door-in to door-out time to less than 30 minutes to reduce FMC time to reperfusion time has been recommended.[40,41]

If transport and revascularization estimates surpass 120 minutes, fibrinolytic therapy should be administered within 30 minutes of arrival at the referring facility. After fibrinolytics, the AHA/ACC recommend 3 management strategies: facilitated PCI, rescue PCI, or pharmacoinvasive PCI. Facilitated PCI involves the administration of fibrinolytics with the intent to immediately transfer to a catheterization laboratory for mechanical reperfusion.[42] Coronary angiography should be delayed 2 hours to 3 hours after fibrinolytic administration, unless there is evidence of ongoing ischemia suggesting fibrinolytics have failed. In those cases, rescue PCI is indicated for emergent mechanical reperfusion in the CCL.[43] Lastly, the pharmacoinvasive strategy involves the use of fibrinolytics followed by a waiting period with plan for revascularization within 24 hours of initial presentation.[44,45] Most centers utilize the approach of primary PCI or facilitated PCI, and the decision is contingent on the availability of transportation and evidence of ongoing ischemia.

Multiple STEMI referrals may occur at tertiary care centers or quaternary care centers, requiring accepting facilities to triage patients who benefit most from early reperfusion with primary PCI or those at highest risk for evolving myocardial infarction. Higher-risk subsets also include those with significant comorbidities, such as left ventricular dysfunction with ejection fraction (EF) less than or equal to 35%, peripheral arterial disease, prior revascularization, ongoing biomarker release after fibrinolytic therapy, increasing amplitude or persistence of ST elevation, and in cardiogenic shock. Patients may experience temporary improvement with fibrinolysis; however, they remain at high risk of reinfarction, recurrent ischemia, new or worsening heart failure, and cardiogenic shock. In the TRANSFER-AMI trial, those treated with facilitated PCI versus standard care (rescue PCI or cardiac catheterization within 2 weeks after randomization) were less likely to experience the composite endpoint of death, reinfarction, recurrent ischemia, new or worsening heart failure, or cardiogenic shock within 30 days of presentation, primarily driven by a reduction in recurrent ischemia and development of new or worsening heart failure.[46] One-third of the standard care group underwent urgent catheterization within 12 hours of fibrinolysis. The use of fibrinolytics in STEMI patients is an effective strategy for those who cannot be transferred to a PCI center in under 120 minutes from FMC and, in rare cases, may be in concordance with a patient's goals of care if they wish to avoid invasive procedures.[47]

Transfer of patients to PCI-capable centers is associated with a mortality benefit.[48] US data suggest that most patients with STEMI who require transfer for primary PCI remain untreated within 120 minutes of FMC, despite the average time for interfacility transport being less than 60 minutes.[48] Prior series have associated reduced delays with a prehospital ECG and ED notification, EMS transport to first hospital versus self-transport, transfer to local rather than nonlocal hospitals, and early transfer activation.[41,49–53]

Interventions that expedite the transfer decision, such as physician access to field ECG and early involvement of a cardiology team, may help streamline the transfer process or even divert EMS to PCI-capable centers, allowing for earlier activation of the CCL at the receiving facility and minimizing ischemic time.[53–59] Patients presenting with acute STEMI and cardiogenic shock may have further delays in care because they require stabilization prior to transport to a PCI-capable center.[60]

Its recommended to transfer STEMI patients to a PCI-capable facility after the administration of fibrinolytics as coronary patency rates vary upon initial angiography.[3] In Gusto-1 and RAPID-2, the angiographic patency of the culprit vessel was between 31% and 61%, depending on the fibrinolytic used.[61–64] The lack of coronary patency is associated with progressive myocardial infarction and the need for revascularization requiring the availability of a CCL. Approximately 50% of cases require rescue PCI.[61–64]

Once transport is arranged, guideline-based STEMI management should ensue while awaiting transport. All patients should receive full-dose, non–enteric-coated aspirin, 325 mg, and a P2Y12 inhibitor, preferably oral ticagrelor (loading dose, 180 mg) or prasugrel (loading dose, 60 mg).[3,65–68] Prasugrel carries a specific boxed warning in the United States for patients with a history of transient ischemic attack/stroke as well as those aged greater than or equal to 75 years, because there is an increased risk of fatal and intracranial bleeding.[34] Clopidogrel, 600 mg, may be used but is not the preferred agent. If fibrinolytics are used as revascularization strategy, a reduced loading dose of

clopidogrel, 300 mg, is indicated for patients less than 75 years old but no loading dose for patients greater than or equal to 75 years old.[3,69] Ticagrelor, 180 mg, has been shown to be safe for patients less than 75 years old after fibrinolytics but has not been included in the guidelines.[38,39] The initial P2Y12 inhibitor may be changed from clopidogrel to another agent greater than or equal to 12 hours after administration of the fibrinolytic.[70,71]

For patients not receiving fibrinolytics, guidelines recommend heparin administration with an initial bolus dose of 70 U/kg to 100 U/kg (maximum 10,000-U bolus). Lower doses, between 50 U/kg and 70 U/kg (maximum 7000-U bolus), are suggested for patients receiving concomitant glycoprotein IIb/IIIa inhibitors.[3] If fibrinolytics are administered, the ACC/AHA guidelines recommend a heparin bolus dose of 60 U/kg, with maximum 4000-U bolus, followed by an infusion rate of 12 U/kg/h, with maximum 1000 U/h.[3] Alternatively, a loading dose of enoxaparin may be administered (<75 years old, 30 mg, IV bolus, followed in 15 minutes by 1 mg/kg, subcutaneously, every 12 hours; ≥75 years old, 0.75 mg/kg, subcutaneously, every 12 hours; maximum, 75 mg, for the first 2 doses).[3]

The choice of fibrinolytic therapy largely is dependent on local availability. For example, streptokinase is not available in the United States or Canada. Tenecteplase is the preferred agent for those transferring requiring fibrinolytic therapy due to its ease of administration, because it requires only 1 dose. Tenecteplase has similar efficacy outcomes to alteplase and reteplase but with a lower rate of noncerebral bleeding events compared with alteplase.[72–74]

Clinical Care Points: Management of Transfer ST Elevation Myocardial Infarction Patients

- Primary PCI should be attempted if a STEMI patient presents to a non–PCI-capable facility and the treating team can achieve a DTBT of less than 120 minutes. If transport and revascularization estimates surpass 120 minutes, fibrinolytic therapy should be administered within 30 minutes of arrival at the referring facility.
- If fibrinolytics are used as the primary revascularization strategy, a reduced loading dose of clopidogrel, 300 mg, is indicated for patients less than 75 years old but no loading dose should be given if greater than or equal to 75 years old. Ticagrelor may be safe in this setting but is not yet approved. In this setting, heparin,

bolus dose of 60 U/kg, with a maximum of 4000 U, followed by an infusion rate, 12 U/kg/h, with a maximum of 1000 U per hour. Alternatively, a loading dose of enoxaparin may be administered (<75 years old: 30-mg, IV bolus, followed in 15 min by 1 mg/kg, subcutaneously, every 12 hours; ≥75 years old: 0.75 mg/kg, subcutaneously, every 12 hours; maximum, 75 mg, for the first 2 doses).

- Tenecteplase is the preferred agent for those requiring fibrinolytic therapy prior to transfer

MANAGEMENT OF IN-HOSPITAL ST ELEVATION MYOCARDIAL INFARCTION

STEMI complicating the hospital course of an admitted patient is a rare but morbid event. The typical anginal symptoms commonly encountered with STEMIs may not be present because patients generally are inactive during hospitalization or may be intubated and/or sedated, limiting their ability to communicate chest pain or anginal equivalents.[24,75] In all patients who complain of chest pain or an anginal equivalent, such as shortness of breath, an immediate ECG must be obtained. In nonverbal, sedated, or intubated patients, objective changes in their hemodynamics, telemetry, or respiratory status should cue an urgent ECG. STEs in the inpatient setting require careful considerations of alternative diagnosis because often they are unrelated to myocardial injury (see Box 1). For example, pericarditis and myocarditis both can result in ST-segment elevation, albeit typically in a diffuse nonterritorial lead pattern with concomitant PR depression. Takotsubo cardiomyopathy may present with STE but is a diagnosis of exclusion and typically requires urgent catheterization to exclude an arterial occlusion. Electrical variants, such as Brugada syndrome or early repolarization, could show elevated J-points on ECG and suspicion of ACS often can be reduced by comparing to prior ECGs. If STEs are present in the right clinical context, immediate consultation with cardiology and CCL activation should follow. In scenarios where the diagnosis remains unclear, bedside echocardiogram to assess for wall motion abnormalities or newly reduced EF may help illuminate the etiology. Due to these factors, those who develop STEMI while hospitalized are a nonuniform group of patients with complex comorbidities and generally have worse outcomes compared with those with classically presenting STEMI.[76,77] A diagnosis of an inpatient STEMI also portends a much greater risk of morbidity and mortality, with a survival rate to discharge of 63.7% versus 96.9%, respectively, for those who present acutely with primary STEMI.[78] Multiple studies have demonstrated a longer time to ECG, time to CCL activation, and time to reperfusion for in-hospital STEMIs.[24,75] The development of rapid response teams may decrease the barriers of obtaining an ECG and can help bring ancillary staff in case of CCL activation. Comorbid conditions add to the higher mortality rate of inpatient STEMIs. In the MITRA registry, inpatients who suffered a myocardial infarction had twice as high mortality rates compared with outpatients with myocardial infarctions (27.3% vs 13.9%, respectively) and were more likely to have recent gastrointestinal bleed (7.2% vs 5.4%, respectively), central nervous system infarction (3% vs 1.2%, respectively), recent surgery (7% vs 1%, respectively), and renal insufficiency (8.2% vs 3.3%, respectively).[76] These comorbidities must be taken into consideration when deciding the reperfusion strategy, antiplatelet agents, and anticoagulation.

Clinical Care Points: Management of In-hospital ST Elevation Myocardial Infarction Patients

- In-hospital patients may not present with typical angina symptoms or they may be unable to communicate their symptoms.
- STEs in the inpatient setting require careful considerations of alternative diagnosis because often they are unrelated to myocardial injury.
- Bedside ECG can assess for wall motion abnormalities or newly reduced EF if diagnosis is unclear.
- Inpatient STEMI patients have a much greater risk of morbidity and mortality with a survival rate to discharge of 63.7% versus 96.9% for those who present acutely with primary STEMI. Longer time to ECG, time to CCL activation, and time to reperfusion contribute to the increased risk.

SUMMARY

Although the overall number of STEMI patients has decreased over recent years, they remain a cornerstone of cardiology management. AHA/ACC guidelines largely focus on time to reperfusion as a key metric, specifically focusing on FMC2D time. After diagnosis, management of STEMI patients is algorithmically driven;

however, physician intuition and experience remain important because these patients are at high risk of decompensation and cardiogenic shock.

DISCLOSURE

The authors have nothing to disclose.

REFERENCES

1. Benjamin EJ, Muntner P, Alonso A, et al. Heart disease and stroke statistics-2019 update: a report from the American Heart Association. Circulation 2019;139(10):e56–528.
2. Desta L, Jernberg T, Löfman I, et al. Incidence, temporal trends, and prognostic impact of heart failure complicating acute myocardial infarction. The SWEDEHEART Registry (Swedish web-system for enhancement and development of evidence-based care in heart disease evaluated according to recomme. JACC Hear Fail 2015;3(3):234–42.
3. O'Gara PT, Kushner FG, Ascheim DD, et al. 2013 ACCF/AHA guideline for the management of st-elevation myocardial infarction: A report of the American college of cardiology foundation/american heart association task force on practice guidelines. J Am Coll Cardiol 2013;61(4):78–140.
4. Thygesen K, Alpert JS, Jaffe AS, et al. Fourth Universal Definition of Myocardial Infarction (2018). Circulation 2018;138(20):e618–51.
5. Ibanez B, James S, Agewall S, et al. 2017 ESC Guidelines for the management of acute myocardial infarction in patients presenting with ST-segment elevation. Eur Heart J 2018;39(2):119–77.
6. Burns E. Posterior Myocardial Infarction • LITFL • ECG Library Diagnosis. 2019. Available at: https://litfl.com/posterior-myocardial-infarction-ecg-library/. Accessed October 30, 2020.
7. Burns E. Right Ventricular Infarction • LITFL • ECG Library Diagnosis. 2019. Available at: https://litfl.com/right-ventricular-infarction-ecg-library/. Accessed October 19, 2020.
8. Jacobs AK, Antman EM, Faxon DP, et al. Development of systems of care for ST-elevation myocardial infarction patients: executive summary. Circulation 2007;116(2):217–30.
9. Ting HH, Krumholz HM, Bradley EH, et al. Implementation and integration of prehospital ECGs into systems of care for acute coronary syndrome: A scientific statement from the American Heart Association Interdisciplinary Council on quality of care and outcomes research, Emergency Cardiovascular Care Committee, Council on cardiovascular nursing, and Council on clinical cardiology. Circulation 2008;118(10):1066–79.
10. Curtis JP, Portnay EL, Wang Y, et al. The Pre-Hospital Electrocardiogram and Time to Reperfusion in Patients With Acute Myocardial Infarction, 2000-2002. Findings From the National Registry of Myocardial Infarction-4. J Am Coll Cardiol 2006;47(8):1544–52.
11. Ortolani P, Marzocchi A, Marrozzini C, et al. Clinical impact of direct referral to primary percutaneous coronary intervention following pre-hospital diagnosis of ST-elevation myocardial infarction. Eur Heart J 2006;27(13):1550–7.
12. Kontos MC, Gunderson MR, Zegre-Hemsey JK, et al. Prehospital Activation of Hospital Resources (PreAct) ST-Segment–Elevation Myocardial Infarction (STEMI): A Standardized Approach to Prehospital Activation and Direct to the Catheterization Laboratory for STEMI Recommendations From the American Heart Association's Mission: Lifeline Program. J Am Heart Assoc 2020;9(2). https://doi.org/10.1161/JAHA.119.011963.
13. Shavadia JS, Roe MT, Chen AY, et al. Association Between Cardiac Catheterization Laboratory Pre-Activation and Reperfusion Timing Metrics and Outcomes in Patients With ST-Segment Elevation Myocardial Infarction Undergoing Primary Percutaneous Coronary Intervention: A Report From the ACTION Registry. JACC Cardiovasc Interv 2018;11(18):1837–47.
14. Hobl EL, Stimpfl T, Ebner J, et al. Morphine decreases clopidogrel concentrations and effects: A randomized, double-blind, placebo-controlled trial. J Am Coll Cardiol 2014;63(7):630–5.
15. Parodi G, Bellandi B, Xanthopoulou I, et al. Morphine is associated with a delayed activity of oral antiplatelet agents in patients with st-elevation acute myocardial infarction undergoing primary percutaneous coronary intervention. Circ Cardiovasc Interv 2015;8(1). https://doi.org/10.1161/CIRCINTERVENTIONS.114.001593.
16. Farag M, Srinivasan M, Gorog D. MORPHINE USE IMPAIRS THROMBOTIC STATUS IN PATIENTS WITH ST-ELEVATION MYOCARDIAL INFARCTION UNDERGOING PRIMARY PERCUTANEOUS CORONARY INTERVENTION. J Am Coll Cardiol 2016;67(13):40.
17. de Waha S, Eitel I, Desch S, et al. Intravenous morphine administration and reperfusion success in ST-elevation myocardial infarction: insights from cardiac magnetic resonance imaging. Clin Res Cardiol 2015;104(9):727–34.
18. Bonin M, Mewton N, Roubille F, et al. Effect and safety of morphine use in acute anterior ST-segment elevation myocardial infarction. J Am Heart Assoc 2018;7(4). https://doi.org/10.1161/JAHA.117.006833.
19. Stub D, Smith K, Bernard S, et al. Air versus oxygen in ST-segment-elevation myocardial infarction. Circulation 2015;131(24):2143–50.

20. Mccaul M, Lourens A, Kredo T. Pre-hospital versus in-hospital thrombolysis for ST-elevation myocardial infarction. Cochrane Database Syst Rev 2014;2014(9). https://doi.org/10.1002/14651858.CD010191.pub2.

21. Morrison LJ, Verbeek PR, McDonald AC, et al. Mortality and prehospital thrombolysis for acute myocardial infarction. A meta-analysis. J Am Med Assoc 2000;283(20):2686–92.

22. Morrow DA, Antman EM, Sayah A, et al. Evaluation of the time saved by prehospital initiation of reteplase for ST-elevation myocardial infarction: Results of the Early Retavase-Thrombolysis In Myocardial Infarction (ER-TIMI) 19 trial. J Am Coll Cardiol 2002;40(1):71–7.

23. Bonnefoy E, Steg PG, Boutitie F, et al. Comparison of primary angioplasty and pre-hospital fibrinolysis in acute myocardial infarction (CAPTIM) trial: a 5-year follow-up. Eur Heart J 2009;30(13):1598–606.

24. Levine GN, Dai X, Henry TD, et al. In-Hospital ST-Segment Elevation Myocardial Infarction: Improving Diagnosis, Triage, and Treatment. JAMA Cardiol 2018;3(6):527–31.

25. Lange DC, Conte S, Pappas-Block E, et al. Cancellation of the cardiac catheterization lab after activation for ST-Segment-Elevation Myocardial Infarction. Circ Cardiovasc Qual Outcomes 2018;11(8):e004464.

26. Wang K, Asinger RW, Marriott HJL. ST-segment elevation in conditions other than acute myocardial infarction. N Engl J Med 2003;349(22):2128–35.

27. Evangelista A, Isselbacher EM, Bossone E, et al. Insights from the international registry of acute aortic dissection: A 20-year experience of collaborative clinical research. Circulation 2018;137(17):1846–60.

28. Montalescot G, Zeymer U, Silvain J, et al. Intravenous enoxaparin or unfractionated heparin in primary percutaneous coronary intervention for ST-elevation myocardial infarction: The international randomised open-label ATOLL trial. Lancet 2011;378(9792):693–703.

29. Silvain J, Beygui F, Barthélémy O, et al. Efficacy and safety of enoxaparin versus unfractionated heparin during percutaneous coronary intervention: Systematic review and meta-analysis. BMJ 2012;344(7844):16.

30. Zeymer U, Arntz HR, Mark B, et al. Efficacy and safety of a high loading dose of clopidogrel administered prehospitally to improve primary percutaneous coronary intervention in acute myocardial infarction: The randomized CIPAMI trial. Clin Res Cardiol 2012;101(4):305–12.

31. Dörler J, Edlinger M, Alber HF, et al. Clopidogrel pre-treatment is associated with reduced in-hospital mortality in primary percutaneous coronary intervention for acute ST-elevation myocardial infarction. Eur Heart J 2011;32(23):2954–61.

32. Montalescot G, Bolognese L, Dudek D, et al. Pretreatment with Prasugrel in Non–ST-Segment Elevation Acute Coronary Syndromes. N Engl J Med 2013;369(11):999–1010.

33. Storey RF, Angiolillo DJ, Patil SB, et al. Inhibitory effects of ticagrelor compared with clopidogrel on platelet function in patients with acute coronary syndromes: The PLATO (PLATelet inhibition and patient Outcomes) PLATELET substudy. J Am Coll Cardiol 2010;56(18):1456–62.

34. Goldenberg MM. Pharmaceutical approval update. P T 2009;34(9):509–12. Available at: https://pubmed.ncbi.nlm.nih.gov/20140113.

35. Montalescot G, van 't Hof AW, Lapostolle F, et al. Prehospital Ticagrelor in ST-Segment Elevation Myocardial Infarction. N Engl J Med 2014;371(11):1016–27.

36. Franchi F, Rollini F, Rivas A, et al. Platelet inhibition with cangrelor and crushed ticagrelor in patients with ST-Segment-Elevation myocardial infarction undergoing primary percutaneous coronary intervention: results of the CANTIC Study. Circulation 2019;139(14):1661–70.

37. Gargiulo G, Esposito G, Avvedimento M, et al. Cangrelor, tirofiban, and chewed or standard prasugrel regimens in patients with ST-Segment-Elevation Myocardial Infarction: Primary Results of the FABOLUS-FASTER Trial. Circulation 2020;142(5):441–54.

38. Berwanger O, Lopes RD, Moia DDF, et al. Ticagrelor Versus Clopidogrel in Patients With STEMI Treated With Fibrinolysis: TREAT Trial. J Am Coll Cardiol 2019;73(22):2819–28.

39. Berwanger O, Nicolau JC, Carvalho AC, et al. Ticagrelor vs clopidogrel after fibrinolytic therapy in patients with st-elevation myocardial infarction a randomized clinical trial. JAMA Cardiol 2018;3(5):391–9.

40. Wang TY, Nallamothu BK, Krumholz HM, et al. Association of door-in to door-out time with reperfusion delays and outcomes among patients transferred for primary percutaneous coronary intervention. JAMA 2011;305(24):2540–7.

41. Lambert LJ, Brown KA, Boothroyd LJ, et al. Transfer of patients with ST-elevation myocardial infarction for primary percutaneous coronary intervention: a province-wide evaluation of "door-in to door-out" delays at the first hospital. Circulation 2014;129(25):2653–60.

42. Brodie BR. Facilitated percutaneous coronary intervention. Heart 2005;91(12):1527–9.

43. Eeckhout E. Rescue percutaneous coronary intervention: does the concept make sense? Heart 2007;93(5):632–8.

44. Helal AM, Shaheen SM, Elhammady WA, et al. Primary PCI versus pharmacoinvasive strategy for ST elevation myocardial infarction. Int J Cardiol Heart Vasc 2018;21:87–93.

45. Sharma V. Pharmaco-invasive strategy: An attractive alternative for management of ST-elevation myocardial infarction when timely primary percutaneous coronary intervention is not feasible. J Postgrad Med 2018;64(2):73–4.

46. Cantor WJ, Fitchett D, Borgundvaag B, et al. Routine Early Angioplasty after Fibrinolysis for Acute Myocardial Infarction. N Engl J Med 2009; 360(26):2705–18.

47. Vallabhajosyula S, Verghese D, Subramaniam AV, et al. Management and outcomes of uncomplicated ST-segment elevation myocardial infarction patients transferred after fibrinolytic therapy. Int J Cardiol 2020. https://doi.org/10.1016/j.ijcard.2020.08.012.

48. Dauerman HL, Bates ER, Kontos MC, et al. Nationwide Analysis of Patients With ST-Segment-Elevation Myocardial Infarction Transferred for Primary Percutaneous Intervention: Findings From the American Heart Association Mission: Lifeline Program. Circ Cardiovasc Interv 2015;8(5). https://doi.org/10.1161/circinterventions.114.002450.

49. Ward MJ, Vogus TJ, Bonnet K, et al. Breaking down walls: a qualitative evaluation of perceived emergency department delays for patients transferred with ST-elevation myocardial infarction. BMC Emerg Med 2020;20(1):60.

50. Ward MJ, Kripalani S, Storrow AB, et al. Timeliness of interfacility transfer for ED patients with ST-elevation myocardial infarction. Am J Emerg Med 2015;33(3):423–9.

51. Clot S, Rocher T, Morvan C, et al. Door-in to door-out times in acute ST-segment elevation myocardial infarction in emergency departments of non-interventional hospitals: A cohort study. Med 2020;99(23):e20434.

52. Rathod KS, Jain AK, Firoozi S, et al. Outcome of inter-hospital transfer versus direct admission for primary percutaneous coronary intervention: An observational study of 25,315 patients with ST-elevation myocardial infarction from the London Heart Attack Group. Eur Hear J Acute Cardiovasc Care 2020. https://doi.org/10.1177/2048872619882340.

53. Shi O, Khan AM, Rezai MR, et al. Factors associated with door-in to door-out delays among ST-segment elevation myocardial infarction (STEMI) patients transferred for primary percutaneous coronary intervention: a population-based cohort study in Ontario, Canada. BMC Cardiovasc Disord 2018; 18(1):204.

54. Jung MS, Kim YW, Lee S, et al. Effect of percutaneous coronary intervention team prenotification based on real time electrocardiogram transmission in interhospital transfer of ST elevation myocardial infarction patients: pilot trial of Preparing Revascularization Effort before Patients. Clin Exp Emerg Med 2020;7(2):114–21.

55. Zeitouni M, Al-Khalidi HR, Roettig ML, et al. Catheterization Laboratory Activation Time in Patients Transferred With ST-Segment-Elevation Myocardial Infarction: Insights From the Mission: Lifeline STEMI Accelerator-2 Project. Circ Cardiovasc Qual Outcomes 2020;13(7):e006204.

56. Anderson LL, French WJ, Peng SA, et al. Direct Transfer From the Referring Hospitals to the Catheterization Laboratory to Minimize Reperfusion Delays for Primary Percutaneous Coronary Intervention: Insights From the National Cardiovascular Data Registry. Circ Cardiovasc Interv 2015; 8(9):e002477.

57. Jollis JG, Al-Khalidi HR, Roettig ML, et al. Impact of Regionalization of ST-Segment-Elevation Myocardial Infarction Care on Treatment Times and Outcomes for Emergency Medical Services-Transported Patients Presenting to Hospitals With Percutaneous Coronary Intervention: Mission: Lifeline Accelerator. Circulation 2018;137(4):376–87.

58. Estévez-Loureiro R, López-Sainz A, Pérez de Prado A, et al. Timely reperfusion for ST-segment elevation myocardial infarction: Effect of direct transfer to primary angioplasty on time delays and clinical outcomes. World J Cardiol 2014;6(6): 424–33.

59. Hung SC, Mou CY, Chan KC, et al. A direct connection promotes time efficiency for transfer of ST-elevation myocardial infarction patients. Rural Remote Heal 2020;20(2):5690.

60. Kochar A, Al-Khalidi HR, Hansen SM, et al. Delays in Primary Percutaneous Coronary Intervention in ST-Segment Elevation Myocardial Infarction Patients Presenting With Cardiogenic Shock. JACC Cardiovasc Interv 2018;11(18):1824–33.

61. de Belder MA. Coronary Disease: Acute myocardial infarction: failed thrombolysis. Heart 2001;85(1): 104–12.

62. Topol EJ. Acute myocardial infarction: thrombolysis. Heart 2000;83(1):122.

63. An International Randomized Trial Comparing Four Thrombolytic Strategies for Acute Myocardial Infarction. N Engl J Med 1993;329(10):673–82.

64. Weaver WD. Results of the RAPID 1 and RAPID 2 thrombolytic trials in acute myocardial infarction. Eur Hear J 1996;17(Suppl E):14–20.

65. Dangas G, Mehran R, Guagliumi G, et al. Role of clopidogrel loading dose in patients with ST-segment elevation myocardial infarction undergoing primary angioplasty: results from the HORIZONS-AMI (harmonizing outcomes with revascularization and stents in acute myocardial infarction) trial. J Am Coll Cardiol 2009;54(15):1438–46.

66. Mehta SR, Tanguay J-F, Eikelboom JW, et al. Double-dose versus standard-dose clopidogrel and high-dose versus low-dose aspirin in individuals undergoing percutaneous coronary intervention for

acute coronary syndromes (CURRENT-OASIS 7): a randomised factorial trial. Lancet 2010;376(9748): 1233–43.

67. Franchi F, Rollini F, Cho JR, et al. Impact of Escalating Loading Dose Regimens of Ticagrelor in Patients With ST-Segment Elevation Myocardial Infarction Undergoing Primary Percutaneous Coronary Intervention: Results of a Prospective Randomized Pharmacokinetic and Pharmacodynamic Investigat. JACC Cardiovasc Interv 2015;8(11):1457–67.

68. Wiviott SD, Braunwald E, McCabe CH, et al. Prasugrel versus Clopidogrel in Patients with Acute Coronary Syndromes. N Engl J Med 2007;357(20):2001–15.

69. Sabatine MS, Cannon CP, Gibson CM, et al. Addition of clopidogrel to aspirin and fibrinolytic therapy for myocardial infarction with ST-segment elevation. N Engl J Med 2005;352(12):1179–89.

70. Angiolillo DJ, Rollini F, Storey RF, et al. International Expert Consensus on Switching Platelet P2Y(12) Receptor-Inhibiting Therapies. Circulation 2017;136(20):1955–75.

71. Franchi F, Faz GT, Rollini F, et al. Pharmacodynamic Effects of Switching From Prasugrel to Ticagrelor: Results of the Prospective, Randomized SWAP-3 Study. JACC Cardiovasc Interv 2016;9(11):1089–98.

72. A comparison of reteplase with alteplase for acute myocardial infarction. N Engl J Med 1997;337(16): 1118–23.

73. Topol EJ, Ohman EM, Armstrong PW, et al. Survival outcomes 1 year after reperfusion therapy with either alteplase or reteplase for acute myocardial infarction: results from the Global Utilization of Streptokinase and t-PA for Occluded Coronary Arteries (GUSTO) III Trial. Circulation 2000;102(15): 1761–5.

74. Van De Werf F, Adgey J, Ardissino D, et al. Single-bolus tenecteplase compared with front-loaded alteplase in acute myocardial infarction: the ASSENT-2 double-blind randomised trial. Lancet 1999;354(9180):716–22.

75. Pande AN, Jacobs AK. In-hospital ST-segment-elevation myocardial infarction an inside-out approach. Circulation 2014;129(11):1193–5.

76. Zahn R, Schiele R, Seidl K, et al. Acute myocardial infarction occurring in versus out of the hospital: patient characteristics and clinical outcome. J Am Coll Cardiol 2000;35(7):1820–6.

77. Maynard C, Lowy E, Rumsfeld J, et al. The Prevalence and Outcomes of In-Hospital Acute Myocardial Infarction in the Department of Veterans Affairs Health System. Arch Intern Med 2006; 166(13):1410–6.

78. Dai X, Bumgarner J, Spangler A, et al. Acute ST-Elevation Myocardial Infarction in Patients Hospitalized for Noncardiac Conditions. J Am Heart Assoc 2013;2(2):e000004.

Anticoagulation in ST-Elevation Myocardial Infarction

Chirag Bavishi, MD, MPH[a,b], J. Dawn Abbott, MD[a,b,*]

KEYWORDS

- Anticoagulation • ST segment elevation myocardial infarction
- Percutaneous coronary intervention • Clinical trials

KEY POINTS

- Anticoagulation is a cornerstone in the management of acute myocardial infarction (MI) and the available options include unfractionated heparin, enoxaparin, fondaparinux, and bivalirudin.
- Each anticoagulant has unique pharmacologic and pharmacodynamic properties that are inherent to the strengths and weaknesses in treatment strategies for acute MI.
- Several randomized controlled trials evaluating various anticoagulation strategies have provided important insights on their comparative efficacy and safety.
- Unfractionated heparin and bivalirudin remain the most used anticoagulation agents.

INTRODUCTION

Anticoagulation is one of the key strategies in pharmacologic management of acute myocardial infarction. In ST-elevation myocardial infarction (STEMI), anticoagulation is used either in conjunction with primary percutaneous coronary intervention (PCI) or fibrinolytic therapy. It is also used in patients who are deemed not eligible for reperfusion therapy. The pathophysiology underlying STEMI most often consists of vulnerable plaque rupture, erosion, or ulceration and subsequent thrombus formation, leading to various degrees of acute vessel occlusion and myocardial ischemia. After atherosclerotic plaque rupture, the thrombogenic core is exposed, triggering platelet activation and aggregation, and coagulation cascades, resulting in intracoronary thrombus formation. Anticoagulation in primary PCI addresses 2 key processes: initial thrombus generation caused by activation of the anticoagulation pathway and secondary thrombin generation caused by vessel injury from coronary balloon angioplasty and stent implantation. In primary PCI, monocyte–platelet aggregates, a measure of platelet activation and inflammation, peaks 2 to 4 hours after stent implantation, a time period most vulnerable for acute stent thrombosis.[1] Hence, the properties of specific anticoagulants, including their duration of effect, potency, and interactions with other pharmacotherapies, are important factors in the management of STEMI. The risk of recurrent ischemic and bleeding events after primary PCI also influences the choice of antithrombotic therapies. In the HORIZONS-AMI trial, after primary PCI, rates for bleeding exceeded those for ischemia within 30 days whereas beyond 30 days, the risk of ischemia exceeded that of bleeding.[2] In addition to the antiplatelet therapy, periprocedural anticoagulation therapies play a vital role in benefit-to-risk ratio of guideline-recommended antithrombotic therapies. Four anticoagulant options are currently available for primary PCI: unfractionated heparin (UFH), enoxaparin, fondaparinux, and bivalirudin (Table 1).

Funding: None.

[a] Lifespan Cardiovascular Institute, Rhode Island Hospital, 593 Eddy Street, Providence, RI 02903, USA; [b] Warren Alpert Medical School at Brown University, 222 Richmond Street, Providence, RI 02903, USA

* Corresponding author. Division of Cardiology, Rhode Island Hospital, Warren Alpert Medical School at Brown University, 814 APC, 593 Eddy Street, Providence, RI.

E-mail address: jabbott@lifespan.org

Table 1
Key characteristics of various anticoagulants used in primary PCI

	UFH	Enoxaparin	Fondaparinux	Bivalirudin
Mechanism of action	Binds to AT, inhibits factor Xa and other proteases	binds to at, inhibits factor xa	Binds to AT, inhibits Factor Xa	Directly binds to thrombin
Factor Xa:IIa inhibition	1:1	3–4:1	Only Xa	Only IIa
Mode of administration	IV	IV, SC	IV, SC	IV
Plasma protein binding	High	Low	None	None
Half-life[a]	~60 min	3–6 h	17–21 h	25 min
Clearance	Reticuloendothelial system and renal	Largely renal	Renal	Enzymatic and Renal
Use in renal failure	No restriction	Contraindicated if eGFR <30	Contraindicated if eGFR <30	Needs dose adjustment and close monitoring
Platelet activation	+++	+	-	-
Reversal agent	Protamine (100%)	Protamine (60%–75%)	None	None
HIT	1%–5%	0.1%–1%	Very rare	None
Usual dose in primary PCI	70–100U/kg bolus without GPIs, 50–70U/kg bolus with GPIs	0.5 mg/kg IV bolus	2.5 mg IV/SC	0.75 mg/kg bolus, 1.75 mg/kg/h infusion
Monitoring	ACT	Anti-Xa, ACT	Anti-Xa	ACT+
Cost	+	+	++	++

Abbreviations: A, antithrombin; ACT, activated clotting time; eGFR, estimated glomerular filtration rate; GP, glycoprotein IIb/IIIa inhibitors; IV, intravenous; SC, subcutaneous; UFH, unfractionated heparin.

[a] At standard doses at normal creatinine clearance, +ACT does not suggest therapeutic effect, only reflects delivery of drug.

UNFRACTIONATED HEPARIN

UFH works as an anticoagulant by inactivating thrombin and activated factor Xa through heparin–antithrombin complex formation (Fig. 1). By inactivating thrombin, heparin prevents fibrin formation and also inhibits thrombin-mediated activation of platelets and coagulation factors V and VIII. The anticoagulant response of UFH is nonlinear, the half-life increases from 30 minutes after an intravenous bolus of 25 U/kg to 60 minutes with a bolus of 100 U/kg and to 150 minutes with a bolus of 400 U/kg. In addition to the heterogenous effects, a lack of ability to bind to clot-bound thrombin, inhibition by platelet factors, and variable patient responses are some of the major limitations.

Heparin has been available since the 1930s; however, there is no placebo-controlled randomized trial of UFH in STEMI. The dosing for UFH has evolved over time, with the evolution in other pharmacotherapies for acute MI. The activated clotting time (ACT) is the most commonly used point-of-care test to monitor UFH during PCI procedures. In a subanalysis

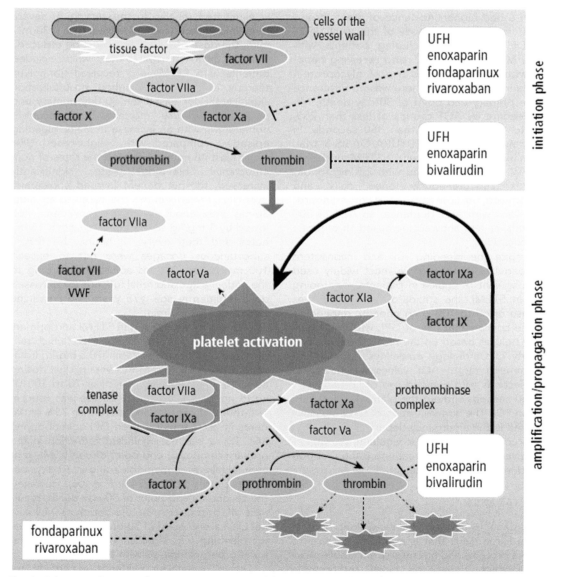

Fig. 1. Schematic diagram of coagulation cascade and the target coagulation factors of anticoagulants used in the management of STEMI. (Figure adapted and modified from Ahrens et al.[28] (with permission).)

of the STEEPLE trial, which includes patients undergoing elective PCI, an ACT of less than 325 seconds was associated with increased ischemic complications.[3] However, in a meta-analysis of 4 randomized controlled trials[4] in patients undergoing PCI, the ACT did not correlate with ischemic complications, although there was a linear increase in bleeding risk as the ACT approached 365 seconds, which leveled off beyond that value. These studies, however, are more than a decade old, included patients with broad indications, used largely aspirin and clopidogrel as antiplatelet agents, and used femoral access for intervention and older generation stents, which a had higher incidence of stent thrombosis. In a recent substudy of the VALIDATE-SWEDEHEART trial[5] including patients with acute MI undergoing PCI and receiving heparin, without the planned use of glycoprotein IIb/IIIa inhibitors (GPI), there was no difference in the primary end point of 30-day death, MI, or bleeding by ACT groups of less than 250, 250 to 350, and more than 350 seconds. In an analysis[6] from the FUTURA/OASIS-8 trial, which included patients with NSTEMI undergoing PCI who were treated with 2.5 mg fondaparinux subcutaneously once daily and randomized to low-dose UFH or standard-dose UFH with ACT guidance, an ACT of 300 seconds or less showed increased thrombotic complications.

Despite the bleeding risk and inconsistent anticoagulation, UFH is the most widely used anticoagulant of choice in patients undergoing PCI. In STEMI, the standard practice involves the use of 60 to 100 U/kg heparin, depending on the concomitant use of GPI, with additional small boluses based on the ACT. The European Society of Cardiology guidelines[7] for NSTEMI recommend target ACT values within 200 to 250 seconds with planned use of GPI and 250 to 350 seconds without the planned use of GPI during PCI. The administration of UFH is usually initiated in the emergency department, whereas bivalirudin and other anticoagulants are generally given in the cardiac catheterization laboratory during the procedure.

ENOXAPARIN

Enoxaparin is a low-molecular-weight heparin derived from UFH that is less likely to bind to plasma proteins and has more predictable pharmacokinetics. Enoxaparin binds antithrombin and inhibits coagulation factors XIa, IXa, Xa, and IIa (thrombin) with greater activity against factor Xa than thrombin. Compared with UFH, the pharmacodynamic profile of enoxaparin has several advantages: reliable anticoagulant effects, thereby eliminating the need for therapeutic monitoring; longer half-life; potential antiplatelet effects via higher degrees of suppression of von Willebrand factor; and a lesser propensity to cause heparin-induced thrombocytopenia. Enoxaparin can be used by intravenous or subcutaneous routes with intravenous route favored owing to its quicker onset of action. After an intravenous bolus of 0.5 mg/kg, a therapeutic level is achieved within minutes and maintained for up to 2 hours. Enoxaparin is metabolized predominantly by the liver and is eliminated renally. In the setting of severe renal impairment (creatinine clearance <30 mL/min), the dose of enoxaparin must be reduced.

In the ExTRACT-TIMI 25 trial,[8] which included patients with STEMI who received fibrinolytic therapy, enoxaparin throughout hospitalization significantly decreased the 30-day primary end point of all-cause mortality and recurrent nonfatal MI, with an increase in major bleeding episodes, compared with weight-based UFH for at least 48 hours. Although the rates of non-intracranial bleeding were significantly increased, the net benefit favored enoxaparin over UFH. Patients in this trial received an initial 30-mg intravenous bolus of enoxaparin, followed by 1 mg/kg subcutaneously within 15 minutes and then every 12 hours; the first 2 subcutaneous dosages were not to exceed 100 mg. The dose was adjusted according to the patient's age and renal function (a decreased dose regimen in age ≥75 years and creatinine clearance <30 mL/min).

The role of enoxaparin in STEMI and primary PCI was studied in the ATOLL trial,[9] which randomized patients to enoxaparin 0.5 mg/kg intravenous bolus at time of PCI versus UFH dosing at 50 to 70 U/kg (if GPI used) or 70 to 100 U/kg (if no GPI used). Radial access was used in two-thirds of patients and more than 75% of patients in both arms received GPI agents during PCI. There was no significant reduction in the primary composite end point of death, MI, procedural failure, or major bleeding at 30 days between 2 arms (28% vs 34%; P = .06). However, the secondary end point of 30-day death, recurrent MI, or urgent revascularization as well as a net clinical end point of 30-day death, MI, or major bleeding was significantly lower in enoxaparin group compared with the UFH group.

Owing to unclear evidence of benefit for enoxaparin over UFH in patients undergoing primary PCI, the 2013 American Heart Association/

American College of Cardiology guidelines[10] do not recommend enoxaparin in primary PCI, whereas the 2017 European Society of Cardiology guidelines[11] provide a class IIa, level of evidence A recommendation for the use of intravenous enoxaparin as an anticoagulation during primary PCI (Table 2).

FONDAPARINUX

Fondaparinux is a selective inhibitor of factor Xa that reversibly binds to antithrombin and rapidly inhibits factor Xa (see Fig. 1). The potential advantages of fondaparinux over UFH include a predictable anticoagulant effect, good bioavailability after subcutaneous injection, daily dosing owing to a long half-life of 15 to 18 hours, and no association with heparin-induced thrombocytopenia. In the OASIS-5 trial,[12] 20,078 patients with NSTEMI were randomized to either fondaparinux 2.5 mg/d or enoxaparin 1 mg/kg twice daily for a mean of 6 days. Fondaparinux was found to be noninferior to enoxaparin in decreasing the risk of ischemic events at 9 days; however, it substantially decreased major bleeding events. In this trial, catheter-related thrombosis occurred more frequently in patients pretreated with fondaparinux (1.3% vs 0.5%; $P = .001$), raising safety concerns and leading to the recommendation to give a bolus of UFH at the time of PCI. The OASIS-6[13] was a complex designed trial that enrolled 12,092 STEMI patients treated either medically or with primary PCI and into 2 strata: fondaparinux versus placebo or fondaparinux versus UFH. Fibrinolytic therapy was used in 45% of patients (mostly in stratum 1), primary PCI was undertaken in 28.9% (mostly in stratum 2), and 23.7% received no reperfusion therapy. The dose of fondaparinux used was 2.5 mg once daily subcutaneously for 8 or fewer days; in patients undergoing primary PCI, fondaparinux

2.5 mg IV bolus was compared with 60 U/kg bolus of UFH followed infusion for 24 to 48 hours. In stratum 2, there was no significant decrease in the primary end point of 30-day death or reinfarction between fondaparinux and UFH (8.3% vs 8.7%; $P = .08$). In patients undergoing primary PCI, there was higher incidence of catheter-related thrombus and coronary complications (abrupt coronary artery closure, new angiographic thrombus, catheter thrombus, no reflow, dissection, or perforation) with fondaparinux. Owing to increased risk for catheter-related thrombosis events, both US and European guidelines give a class III recommendation (harm) for use of fondaparinux alone in primary PCI.[10,11]

BIVALIRUDIN

Bivalirudin, a synthetic analogue of naturally occurring hirudine, is a direct thrombin inhibitor, thereby preventing the conversion of fibrinogen to fibrin (see Fig. 1). Unlike other anticoagulants, its action does not depend on plasma cofactors for inhibition of thrombin generation. The bivalirudin–thrombin bonds are gradually cleaved by thrombin itself, rendering a short half-life of 25 minutes. The potential advantages of bivalirudin include a predictable anticoagulation effect owing to the absence of binding to plasma proteins, a short half-life with a rapid offset in the event of bleeding, the ability to bind to circulating as well as clot bound thrombin, a lack of platelet activation, a low immunogenic potential, and that it does not cause heparin-induced thrombocytopenia. Despite the theoretic advantages of bivalirudin, the clinical evidence comparing bivalirudin and UFH has been equivocal.

Bivalirudin has been studied in several randomized trials of primary PCI (Table 3).[14–19] The HEAT-PPCI trial[14] was an open-label,

Table 2		
Summary of US and European guidelines on anticoagulation in STEMI and primary PCI		
	2013 American Heart Asscoiation/ American College of Cardiology Guidelines	2017 European Society of Cardiology Guidelines
UFH	Class I, LOE C	Class I, LOE C
Enoxaparin	No specific recommendation	Class IIa, LOE A
Fondaparinux	Class III, LOE B	Class III, LOE B
Bivalirudin	Class I, LOE B Class IIa, LOE B[a]	Class IIa, LOE A Class I, LOE C+

[a] Recommendation for bivalirudin monotherapy use compared with UFH and GPI in patients with a high risk of bleeding; +In patients with heparin-induced thrombocytopenia.

Table 3
Summary of key randomized controlled trials comparing bivalirudin with UFH in primary PCI

Trial	Year	Patients	Treatment Arms	GPI Use Bivalirudin	GPI Use UFH	Women	Radial	Primary End Point	NACE	Major Bleeding	ST
HORIZONS-AMI	2007	3602	Bivalirudin vs UFH + GPI	Bailout, 7.5%	Routine, 97.7%	23%	6%	NACE (all-cause death, MI, TVR, stroke or major bleeding); major bleeding	↓	↓	↑
EUROMAX	2013	2198	Bivalirudin vs UFH	Bailout, 7.9%	Routine or bailout, 84%	24%	47%	NACE (all-cause death or major bleeding)	↓	↓	↑
HEAT-PPCI	2014	1812	Bivalirudin vs UFH	Bailout, 13.5%	Bailout, 15.5%	28%	81%	All-cause mortality, stroke, MI, unplanned TLR; major bleeding	↑	↔	↑
BRIGHT (STEMI)	2015	2194[a]	Bivalirudin vs UFH (vs UFH + GPI)[b]	Bailout, 4.6%	Bailout, 5.6%	27%	69%	NACE (all-cause death, MI, TVR, stroke or bleeding)	↓	↓	↔
MATRIX (STEMI)	2015	4010[a]	Bivalirudin vs UFH	Bailout, 6%	Routine or bailout, 4.3%	23%	50%	NACE (all-cause death, MI, stroke or bleeding)	↔	↓	↔
VALIDATE-SWEDEHEART (STEMI)	2017	3005[a]	Bivalirudin vs UFH	Bailout, 1.3%	Bailout, 0.7%	28%	91%	NACE (all-cause death, MI or major bleeding)	↔	↔	↔

Abbreviations: GPI, glycoprotein IIb/IIIa inhibitors; MI, myocardial infarction; NACE, net adverse cardiovascular events; ST, stent thrombosis; TLR, target-lesion revascularization; TVR, target-vessel revascularization; UFH, unfractionated heparin.
[a] Sample size for STEMI group.
[b] For outcomes and GPI use, bivalirudin versus heparin monotherapy group is chosen.

single-center trial of 1812 patients with primary PCI randomized to bivalirudin (bolus of 0.75 mg/kg followed by infusion of 1.75 mg/kg/h for the duration of the procedure) or UFH (bolus dose of 70 U/kg before the procedure with additional doses). The primary outcome of all-cause mortality, stroke, reinfarction, or unplanned target lesion revascularization at 28 days was significantly higher in the bivalirudin group compared with UFH group (8.7% vs 5.7%; P = .01), with no increased risk of major bleeding events. In the HORIZONS-AMI trial,[15] 3602 patients presenting with STEMI were randomized to receive either UFH (bolus dose of 60 U/kg before the procedure with additional doses) plus GPI (abciximab or eptifibatide) or bivalirudin (bolus of 0.75 mg/kg followed by infusion of 1.75 mg/kg/h for the duration of the procedure). At 30 days, the bivalirudin group had a significantly lower rate of net adverse clinical events (9.2% vs 12.1%; P = .005), owing to a lower rate of major bleeding (4.9% vs 8.3%; P < .001), with similar rates of major adverse cardiovascular events (5.4% vs 5.5%; P = .95). Interestingly, an increase in the rate of acute stent thrombosis was noted in the bivalirudin group, which in another post hoc analysis was more frequent in shorter (<45 minutes), procedures likely owing of the rapid offset of bivalirudin's antithrombotic effect during a window of limited oral antiplatelet action.[20] In the EUROMAX trial,[16] 2218 patients with STEMI were randomized to bivalirudin (bolus of 0.75 mg/kg followed by infusion of 1.75 mg/kg/h continued for at least 4 hours after the procedure) or heparin with optional GPI (100 IU/kg without a GPI or 60 IU/kg with a GPI) or an intravenous bolus of enoxaparin (0.5 mg/kg). Compared with controls, the bivalirudin group has a significantly decreased risk of 30-day death or major bleeding (5.1% vs 8.5%; P = .001), as well as 30-day death, reinfarction, or major bleeding (6.6% vs 9.2%; P = .02). These results were largely driven by a substantial decrease in major bleeding. As in the HORIZONS-AMI trial, higher rates of acute stent thrombosis were seen in the bivalirudin group. It is important to note that these trials varied in terms of some important clinical factors, such as the use of pre- and/or post-PCI bivalirudin, use of GPI, dosages and regimen of P2Y12 inhibitors, and the access site used for PCI.

The most contemporary trials comparing UFH and bivalirudin are the MATRIX[18] and the VALI-DATE-SWEDEHEART[19] trials. The MATRIX trial[18] randomly assigned 7213 patients with an acute coronary syndrome (56% with STEMI)

undergoing PCI to either bivalirudin or UFH with provisional GPI. The dose for UFH was 70 to 100 U/kg in patients not receiving GPI and a dose of 50 to 70 U/kg in patients receiving GPI, whereas the dose for bivalirudin was a 0.75 mg/kg bolus followed by an infusion of 1.75 mg/kg/h for the duration of the PCI. The primary end point was 30-day major adverse cardiovascular events (a composite of death, MI, or stroke) and net adverse clinical events (a composite of major bleeding or a major adverse cardiovascular event). In the overall cohort, there was no significant difference in major adverse cardiovascular events or net adverse clinical events between the 2 groups.[18] The rate of definite stent thrombosis was significantly higher in the bivalirudin group (1.0% vs 0.6%; P = .048). Bleeding rates, including major bleeding, was significantly decreased with bivalirudin; however surprisingly, bivalirudin also decreased all-cause and cardiovascular mortality. In the STEMI cohort,[21] there was no significant difference in the primary end points, although the all-cause mortality was marginally better (2.1% vs 3.1%; P = .05); bivalirudin had fewer major bleeding events (1.7% vs 2.8%; P = .02), but had higher rates of definite stent thrombosis (1.3% vs 0.7%; P = .06).

The VALIDATE-SWEDEHEART trial[19] compared UFH monotherapy and bivalirudin in 6005 patients with acute MI (50% STEMI) undergoing PCI, receiving treatment with a potent P2Y12 inhibitor (ticagrelor, prasugrel, or cangrelor) without the planned use of a GPI. The heparin regimen was up to 5000 U intravenous bolus in the emergency room or up to 3000 U intra-arterial in the cardiac catheterization laboratory before angiography, followed by additional doses to make a total dose of 70 to 100 U/kg. The bivalirudin dose was an intravenous bolus of 0.75 mg/kg followed by infusion of 1.75 mg/kg/h. Continuation of the bivalirudin infusion after PCI until completion of the last vial was strongly recommended. The primary end point was all-cause mortality, reinfarction, or major bleeding at 6 months. In this trial, the majority of the patients had radial access (90%), were treated with ticagrelor (95%), and the use of a rescue GPI was minimal (2.4% in the bivalirudin group vs 2.8% in the heparin group). In the overall cohort, there were no differences between UFH and bivalirudin for the primary end point, any of the individual components, or stent thrombosis at 30 days or 6 months.[19] In the STEMI cohort,[22] the rate of the primary end point at 6 months (12.5% vs 13%; P = .64) as well as major bleeding rates (5.1% vs 4.8% at

30 days; 8% vs 8.3% at 6 months) and definite stent thrombosis (2.3% vs 1.9% at 30 days; 2.8% vs 2.6% at 6 months) were similar between the bivalirudin and the UFH groups.

Bivalirudin may have a differential effect in men and women. In a prespecified subgroup analysis from the VALIDATE-SWEDEHEART trial, bivalirudin was associated with a lower risk of primary outcome of mortality, reinfarction, or major bleeding compared with UFH in women, primarily owing to a significant decrease in bleeding events.[23] However, in the MATRIX trial, the rates of major and net adverse cardiac events were not significantly lower with bivalirudin than with UFH in both sexes.[24] Patients with chronic kidney disease, especially in the advanced stages, represents another group at high risk for bleeding and ischemic events. In an analysis from the NCDR CathPCI registry of 71,675 patients with end-stage renal disease undergoing PCI who received monotherapy with either bivalirudin or UFH, patients receiving bivalirudin had significant lower rates of in-hospital bleeding (7.0% vs 9.5%; adjusted odds ratio, 0.82 [0.76–0.87]) and in-hospital mortality (2.6% vs 4.2%; adjusted odds ratio, 0.87 [0.78–0.97]).[25] However, in the HORIZONS-AMI trial, there was no benefit of bivalirudin compared with UFH plus GPI in patients with chronic kidney disease.[26] Because most of the trials either excluded or had only small number of patients with advanced chronic kidney disease, contemporary data are lacking.

Currently, UFH remains the preferred anticoagulant in patients undergoing primary PCI. The initial enthusiasm of decreased bleeding with bivalirudin faded away after the results of the MATRIX and VALIDAE-SWEDEHEART trials were published. The increased rates of acute stent thrombosis, marginal benefit over heparin monotherapy for bleeding events when radial access is used, and significant higher cost are the main factors preventing the widespread adoption of bivalirudin. With the increasing use of radial access for primary PCI, lower use of GPI, and use of potent P2Y12 inhibitors, the incremental benefit of bivalirudin over UFH monotherapy remains uncertain. However, a recent patient-level meta-analysis[27] of 8 randomized controlled trials including 27,409 patients (55% STEMI) comparing bivalirudin with UFH showed interesting findings. In the overall cohort, there was no difference in ischemic end points; however, in patients with STEMI (n = 15,254), bivalirudin decreased the 30-day cardiac mortality (2.1% vs 2.7%) and serious bleeding events (3.5% vs 6%), despite there being higher rates of MI

(2.4% vs 1.7%) and stent thrombosis (1.7% vs 1.2%). The mortality benefit was pronounced in patients treated with post-PCI high-dose bivalirudin infusion, which mitigated the MI and stent thrombosis risk.[27] These results concerning lower mortality and bleeding with bivalirudin in STEMI are intriguing; however, it remains to be seen if they are compelling enough to change the guidelines. With no major randomized controlled trial on horizon, it is unlikely to have further data on optimal anticoagulation in primary PCI.

Currently, we have 3 potential options for anticoagulation during primary PCI: (1) UFH monotherapy with provisional or bailout use of GPI, (2) bivalirudin with bailout use of GPI, and, (3) UFH and routine GPI (least preferred). UFH monotherapy and bivalirudin with post-PCI infusion remains the 2 most viable options. Our preferred anticoagulation strategy is UFH 100U/kg with additional boluses based on ACT values, with the goal ACT of greater than 250 seconds. The use of GPI is only considered as an adjunct in the setting of heavy thrombus burden. On a case-by-case basis, bivalirudin is considered particularly when femoral access is used for primary PCI.

CLINICS CARE POINTS

- Currently, unfractionated heparin with provisional or bailout use of a glycoprotein IIb/IIIa inhibitor is the most common anticoagulation strategy.

- The use of glycoprotein IIb/IIIa inhibitors can be considered as an adjunct to anticoagulation in the setting of percutaneous coronary intervention (PCI) with inadequate P2Y12 pretreatment, heavy thrombus burden or no reflow.

- Owing to increased risk for catheter-related thrombosis events, Fondaparinux should not be used as the sole anticoagulant in patients undergoing PCI.

- Bivalirudin can be beneficial in patients at high bleeding risk, particularly when femoral access is used, and post-PCI infusion of bivalirudin should be strongly considered to mitigate the stent thrombosis risk.

ACKNOWLEDGMENTS

None.

CONFLICTS OF INTERESTS/DISCLOSURES

The authors have no conflicts of interest to declare.

REFERENCES

1. Michelson AD, Barnard MR, Krueger LA, et al. Circulating monocyte-platelet aggregates are a more sensitive marker of in vivo platelet activation than platelet surface P-selectin: studies in baboons, human coronary intervention, and human acute myocardial infarction. Circulation 2001;104(13): 1533–7.
2. Giustino G, Mehran R, Dangas GD, et al. Characterization of the average daily ischemic and bleeding risk after primary PCI for STEMI. J Am Coll Cardiol 2017;70(15):1846–57.
3. Montalescot G, Cohen M, Salette G, et al. Impact of anticoagulation levels on outcomes in patients undergoing elective percutaneous coronary intervention: insights from the STEEPLE trial. Eur Heart J 2008;29(4):462–71.
4. Brener SJ, Moliterno DJ, Lincoff AM, et al. Relationship between activated clotting time and ischemic or hemorrhagic complications: analysis of 4 recent randomized clinical trials of percutaneous coronary intervention. Circulation 2004;110(8):994–8.
5. Sharma T, Rylance R, Karlsson S, et al. Relationship between degree of heparin anticoagulation and clinical outcome in patients receiving potent P2Y12-inhibitors with no planned glycoprotein IIb/IIIa inhibitor during percutaneous coronary intervention in acute myocardial infarction: a VALIDATE-SWEDEHEART substudy. Eur Heart J Cardiovasc Pharmacother 2020;6(1):6–13.
6. Ducrocq G, Jolly S, Mehta SR, et al. Activated clotting time and outcomes during percutaneous coronary intervention for non-ST-segment-elevation myocardial infarction: insights from the FUTURA/OASIS-8 Trial. Circ Cardiovasc Interv 2015;8(4): e002044.
7. Roffi M, Patrono C, Collet JP, et al. 2015 ESC Guidelines for the management of acute coronary syndromes in patients presenting without persistent ST-segment elevation: Task Force for the Management of Acute Coronary Syndromes in Patients Presenting without Persistent ST-Segment Elevation of the European Society of Cardiology (ESC). Eur Heart J 2016;37(3):267–315.
8. Antman EM, Morrow DA, McCabe CH, et al. Enoxaparin versus unfractionated heparin with fibrinolysis for ST-elevation myocardial infarction. N Engl J Med 2006;354(14):1477–88.
9. Montalescot G, Zeymer U, Silvain J, et al. Intravenous enoxaparin or unfractionated heparin in primary percutaneous coronary intervention for ST-elevation myocardial infarction: the international randomised open-label ATOLL trial. Lancet 2011; 378(9792):693–703.
10. O'Gara PT, Kushner FG, Ascheim DD, et al. 2013 ACCF/AHA guideline for the management of ST-elevation myocardial infarction: executive summary: a report of the American College of Cardiology Foundation/American Heart Association Task Force on Practice Guidelines. J Am Coll Cardiol 2013;61(4):485–510.
11. Ibanez B, James S, Agewall S, et al. 2017 ESC Guidelines for the management of acute myocardial infarction in patients presenting with ST-segment elevation: the Task Force for the management of acute myocardial infarction in patients presenting with ST-segment elevation of the European Society of Cardiology (ESC). Eur Heart J 2018;39(2):119–77.
12. Fifth Organization to Assess Strategies in Acute Ischemic Syndromes I, Yusuf S, Mehta SR, Susan C, et al. Comparison of fondaparinux and enoxaparin in acute coronary syndromes. N Engl J Med 2006;354(14):1464–76.
13. Yusuf S, Mehta SR, Chrolavicius S, et al. Effects of fondaparinux on mortality and reinfarction in patients with acute ST-segment elevation myocardial infarction: the OASIS-6 randomized trial. JAMA 2006;295(13):1519–30.
14. Shahzad A, Kemp I, Mars C, et al. Unfractionated heparin versus bivalirudin in primary percutaneous coronary intervention (HEAT-PPCI): an open-label, single centre, randomised controlled trial. Lancet 2014;384(9957):1849–58.
15. Stone GW, Witzenbichler B, Guagliumi G, et al. Bivalirudin during primary PCI in acute myocardial infarction. N Engl J Med 2008;358(21):2218–30.
16. Steg PG, van 't Hof A, Hamm CW, et al. Bivalirudin started during emergency transport for primary PCI. N Engl J Med 2013;369(23):2207–17.
17. Han Y, Guo J, Zheng Y, et al. Bivalirudin vs heparin with or without tirofiban during primary percutaneous coronary intervention in acute myocardial infarction: the BRIGHT randomized clinical trial. JAMA 2015;313(13):1336–46.
18. Valgimigli M, Frigoli E, Leonardi S, et al. Bivalirudin or unfractionated heparin in acute coronary syndromes. N Engl J Med 2015;373(11):997–1009.
19. Erlinge D, Omerovic E, Frobert O, et al. Bivalirudin versus heparin monotherapy in myocardial infarction. N Engl J Med 2017;377(12):1132–42.
20. Tamez H, Pinto DS, Kirtane AJ, et al. Effect of short procedural duration with bivalirudin on increased risk of acute stent thrombosis in patients with STEMI: a secondary analysis of the HORIZONS-AMI randomized clinical trial. JAMA Cardiol 2017;2(6):673–7.
21. Leonardi S, Frigoli E, Rothenbuhler M, et al. Bivalirudin or unfractionated heparin in patients with acute coronary syndromes managed invasively

with and without ST elevation (MATRIX): randomised controlled trial. BMJ 2016;354:i4935.

22. James S, Andersson J, Angerås O, et al. A randomized trial of Bivalirudin versus Heparin Monotherapy. The STEMI cohort. Denver (CO): TCT; 2017.

23. Venetsanos D, Sederholm Lawesson S, Frobert O, et al. Sex-related response to bivalirudin and unfractionated heparin in patients with acute myocardial infarction undergoing percutaneous coronary intervention: a subgroup analysis of the VALIDATE-SWEDEHEART trial. Eur Heart J Acute Cardiovasc Care 2019;8(6):502–9.

24. Gargiulo G, da Costa BR, Frigoli E, et al. Impact of sex on comparative outcomes of bivalirudin versus unfractionated heparin in patients with acute coronary syndromes undergoing invasive management: a pre-specified analysis of the MATRIX trial. EuroIntervention 2019;15(3):e269–78.

25. Washam JB, Kaltenbach LA, Wojdyla DM, et al. Anticoagulant use among patients with end-stage renal disease undergoing percutaneous coronary intervention: an analysis from the National Cardiovascular Data Registry. Circ Cardiovasc Interv 2018;11(2):e005628.

26. Saltzman AJ, Stone GW, Claessen BE, et al. Long-term impact of chronic kidney disease in patients with ST-segment elevation myocardial infarction treated with primary percutaneous coronary intervention: the HORIZONS-AMI (Harmonizing Outcomes With Revascularization and Stents in Acute Myocardial Infarction) trial. JACC Cardiovasc Interv 2011;4(9):1011–9.

27. Stone GW, Erlinge D, Valgimigli M, et al. Individual patient data pooled analysis of randomized trials of bivalirudin versus heparin in acute myocardial infarction. Presented on October 14, 2020 at TCT 2020. Virtual Meeting.

28. Ahrens I, Bode C, Zirlik A. Anticoagulation during and after acute coronary syndrome. Hamostaseologie 2014;34(1):72–7.

Aspiration Thrombectomy

Matthew C. Evans, MD, Anbukarasi Maran, MD*

KEYWORDS

- Thrombus • Embolization • Microvasculature

KEY POINTS

- Distal embolization of thrombus in ST-segment myocardial infarction is associated with microvascular dysfunction and worsened clinical outcomes.
- Aspiration thrombectomy can help improve percutaneous coronary intervention by allowing for better visualization of target lesion, which allows for better determination of optimal stent size and length.
- Large multicenter randomized controlled trials have failed to demonstrate net clinical benefit from the routine use of aspiration thrombectomy in ST-segment myocardial infarction.
- In patients with high thrombus burden who do not respond to balloon predilation, the use of manual aspiration thrombectomy as a bailout treatment strategy can be considered.

BACKGROUND

ST-segment myocardial infarction (STEMI) is commonly associated with atherosclerotic plaque rupture and occlusion of the coronary artery with thrombus. Over the last 2 decades, primary percutaneous coronary intervention (PCI) has been shown to be superior to fibrinolysis as a means for rapidly achieving reperfusion to the affected artery. Decreased coronary blood flow after PCI is associated with reperfusion injury, which can lead to arrhythmias, contractile dysfunction, microvascular impairment, and irreversible myocardial damage, which in turn can be associated with heart failure and death.[1] Increased thrombus burden during PCI has been associated with increased mortality and adverse outcomes; in an analysis of 812 consecutive patients presenting with STEMI, large as compared with small thrombus burden patients had higher 1-year mortality (12.9% vs 7.8%; $P = .025$) and higher rates of stent thrombosis (8.2% vs 1.3%; $P = .001$).[2] Although PCI remains very effective for restoring epicardial flow of the affected artery, distal embolization of thrombus and the presence of microvascular dysfunction is thought to account for much of the variability in clinical outcomes after the procedure.[3] In a study of 173 consecutive patients who underwent PCI for acute MI, in which 94% achieved restoration of Thrombolysis in Myocardial Infarction (TIMI)-3 coronary flow, only 29.4% of patients had normal myocardial perfusion, as assessed by myocardial blush (contrast opacification of the myocardial bed subtended by the infarct artery). Survival was strongly dependent on the myocardial perfusion grade; the 1-year mortality in patients with normal myocardial blush was 6.8% versus 13.2% among those with decreased myocardial blush and 18.3% in those with absent myocardial blush ($P = .004$).[4]

Coronary thrombectomy offers several potential benefits during PCI. Perhaps most important, thrombectomy may prevent distal embolization and improve microvascular perfusion after the procedure. In addition, thrombectomy in STEMI can allow for better visualization of the target lesion, which can be useful for determining optimal stent size and length. Removal of the thrombus may also prevent late stent malapposition and residual thrombus at the culprit lesion serve as a nidus for stent thrombosis.

There are 2 types of coronary thrombectomy—manual aspiration and mechanical rheolytic thrombectomy. Manual aspiration devices

---

Division of Cardiology, Medical University of South Carolina, 30 Courtenay Drive, 326/MSC 592, Charleston, SC 29425, USA
* Corresponding author.
E-mail address: maran@musc.edu

Intervent Cardiol Clin 10 (2021) 317–322
https://doi.org/10.1016/j.iccl.2021.04.001

are significantly less expensive and easier to use, and thus are far more commonly used in clinical practice. These devices consist of a tapered microcatheter with a guidewire and aspiration lumen attached to a syringe, whereas the mechanical thrombectomy devices (such as the AngioJet Ultra thrombectomy system; Boston Scientific, Marlborough, MA) have active mechanical suction and high-velocity saline jets to break up and remove the thrombus.

Common clinical scenarios where aspiration thrombectomy is thought to be less successful include bifurcation lesions, heavily calcified lesions, and tortuous coronary arteries, and newer generation aspiration catheters have achieved improved deliverability in these instances with the introduction of a stylet-based system.[5] Although uncommon in the hands of experienced operators, the 2 most significant complications of aspiration thrombectomy are dissection of the coronary artery and thrombus dislodgement during retrieval leading to the embolization of a nonculprit vessel.[6]

DISCUSSION

Much of the initial enthusiasm regarding the use of routine aspiration thrombectomy in STEMI came from the Thrombus Aspiration during Percutaneous Coronary Intervention in Acute Myocardial Infarction Study (TAPAS), which was a single-center, prospective, randomized trial where 1071 patients presenting with STEMI were randomized to undergo treatment with either thrombus aspiration or conventional PCI before undergoing coronary angiography. The primary end point was a myocardial blush score of 0 or 1, defined as absent or minimal myocardial blush. Secondary end points were the postprocedural restoration of TIMI-3 flow, complete resolution of ST-segment elevation, target vessel revascularization, reinfarction, death, and the combination of major adverse cardiac events by 30 days after randomization. Retrieved aspirated material was sent for histopathologic examination, and atheroembolic material was retrieved in 73% of patients who underwent aspiration thrombectomy.

With respect to the primary end point, a myocardial blush grade of 0 or 1 occurred in 84 of the 490 patients (17.1%) in the aspiration thrombectomy group and in 129 of the 490 patients (26.3%) in the conventional therapy group ($P<.001$). Patients in the aspiration thrombectomy group had higher rates of complete ST-segment resolution (56.6% vs 44.2%; $P<.001$) and were less likely to develop

pathologic Q waves on their EKG (15.9% vs 24.5%; $P = .001$).

There was no significant difference between the 2 groups in the incidence of major bleeding (3.8% vs 3.4%; $P = .11$), death (2.1% vs 4.0%; $P = .07$), reinfarction (0.8% vs 1.9%; $P = .11$), target vessel revascularization (4.5% vs 5.8%; $P = .34$), or 30-day major adverse cardiac events (6.8% vs 9.4%; $P = .12$), but the rates of death and major adverse cardiac events at 30 days were both significantly related to myocardial blush grade and resolution of ST-segment elevation. The 30-day mortality with a myocardial blush grade of 0 or 1, 2, and 3 was 5.2%, 2.9%, and 1.0%, respectively ($P = .003$).[7] Although TAPAS was underpowered for hard clinical end points, in a follow-up 1-year analysis, death from cardiovascular causes was lower in the aspiration thrombectomy group compared with conventional PCI (3.6% vs 6.7%; $P = .02$).[8]

After the publication of TAPAS, subsequent practice guidelines were changed to recommend the routine use of manual aspiration thrombectomy in STEMI.[9,10] Shortly thereafter, a meta-analysis of 17 smaller randomized trials (a total of 3909 patients) demonstrated not only no difference in 30-day mortality (2.3% vs 2.6%; $P = .42$) among patients randomized to undergo thrombectomy compared with conventional PCI, but thrombectomy was also associated with a greater risk of stroke (1.0% vs 0.2%; $P = .04$). There was a trend toward lower mortality with manual aspiration compared with mechanical thrombectomy devices.[11]

Another subsequent meta-analysis of 2686 patients enrolled in 11 trials demonstrated a decrease in all-cause mortality with thrombectomy compared with PCI alone ($P = .049$). In this study, patients randomized to undergo thrombectomy in the subgroup that received glycoprotein IIb/IIIa inhibitors experienced a further survival benefit ($P = .045$) suggesting thrombectomy may provide an additional effect particularly in those with high thrombus burden.[12]

In another meta-analysis of 6415 patients in 30 studies, manual aspiration thrombectomy was associated with a decrease in mortality with a mean follow-up of 5 months (2.7% vs 4.4%; $P = .018$), whereas mechanical thrombectomy was associated with an increase in mortality (5.3% vs 2.8%; $P = .050$) compared with PCI alone. There was no significant difference in the risk of stroke with either device ($P = .085$ for aspiration thrombectomy and $P = .14$ for mechanical thrombectomy).[13]

In a head-to-head comparison between the 2 proposed strategies to limit distal embolization of thrombus in STEMI, manual aspiration thrombectomy and intracoronary abciximab, a glycoprotein IIb/IIIa inhibitor, were studied in the Intracoronary Abciximab and Aspiration Thrombectomy in Patients with Large Anterior Myocardial Infarction (INFUSE-AMI) trial. There were 452 patients presenting with STEMI owing to proximal or mid left anterior descending artery occlusion who were randomized to undergo primary PCI in a 2 × 2 factorial design to receive intracoronary abciximab delivered locally at the infarct lesion site versus no abciximab and to manual aspiration thrombectomy versus no thrombectomy. The primary end point was infarct size (measured as a percentage of total left ventricular mass) at 30 days assessed by cardiac magnetic resonance imaging. Patients randomized to intracoronary abciximab versus no abciximab had a significant decrease in 30-day infarct size (P = .03). Those randomized to aspiration thrombectomy versus no thrombectomy had no significant different in infarct size at 30 days.[14]

Given the conflicting evidence between TAPAS and these meta-analyses, the Thrombus Aspiration in ST-Elevation Myocardial Infarction in Scandinavia (TASTE) trial was designed to better assess the clinical outcomes associated with routine use of aspiration thrombectomy in STEMI. In TASTE, 7244 patients with STEMI undergoing PCI were randomized to manual thrombus aspiration followed by PCI or conventional PCI alone. The primary end point was all-cause mortality at 30 days.

There was no statistically significant difference in the incidence of 30-day all-cause mortality (2.8% vs 3.0%; P = .63) between the 2 groups. In addition, there was similarly no difference in each of the major secondary end points, namely, repeat hospitalization owing to reinfarction (0.5% vs 0.9%; P = .09), stent thrombosis (P = .06), target lesion revascularization (P = .16), and target vessel revascularization (P = .27).[15] Importantly, there was no significant difference in the rate of stroke or neurologic complications (P = .87) or perforation or tamponade (P = .85).

In a subsequent follow-up 1-year analysis of TASTE, the incidence of death from any cause did not differ between the aspiration thrombectomy and conventional PCI groups (5.3% vs 5.6%; P = .57). There was similarly no difference in the rates of rehospitalization for MI (P = .81), stent thrombosis (P = .51), or a composite of all 3 outcomes (P = .48). These results were consistent across all major prespecified subgroups, including grade of thrombus burden and coronary flow before PCI.[16]

After the publication of TASTE, an updated meta-analysis that included 11,321 patients enrolled from 20 randomized controlled trials was published that demonstrated a composite outcome of major adverse cardiac events was lower in the aspiration thrombectomy arm compared with PCI alone (P = .006). Although all-cause mortality was similar between the groups, late mortality (6–12 months) and the rate of stent thrombosis were significantly lower (P = .021).[17]

To better establish the efficacy of aspiration thrombectomy, the Trial of Routine Aspiration Thrombectomy with PCI versus PCI Alone in Patients with STEMI (TOTAL) was designed to randomize 10,732 patients to undergo PCI with upfront manual aspiration thrombectomy versus PCI alone. The primary outcome was a composite of death from cardiovascular causes, recurrent MI, cardiogenic shock, or New York Heart Association functional class IV heart failure within 180 days. The key safety outcome was stroke within 30 days.

In TOTAL, aspiration thrombectomy improved ST-segment resolution and decreased the rate of distal embolization, but there was no difference in the primary end point between those that underwent thrombectomy and PCI compared with PCI alone (6.9% vs 7.0%; P = 0.86). The rates of cardiovascular death (3.1% vs 3.5%; P = .34) and the primary outcome plus stent thrombosis or target vessel revascularization (9.9% vs 9.8%; P = .95) were also similar. The majority of patients (78.4%) had a high thrombus burden, as defined by TIMI thrombus grade 4 or 5, with similar proportions between both groups. With respect to the key safety outcome, patients undergoing thrombectomy had a higher incidence of stroke (0.7% vs 0.3%; P = .02) compared with PCI alone.[18]

In a subgroup analysis of TOTAL patients with TIMI thrombus grade 3 or greater, there was no difference in the primary outcome—a composite of cardiovascular death, MI, cardiogenic shock, or heart failure—between patients that underwent thrombectomy and those that received conventional PCI in the high or low thrombus burden groups (8.1% vs 8.3%; P = .41). Among those with a high thrombus burden, there was an increased incidence of stroke at 30 days with aspiration thrombectomy compared with PCI alone (0.7% vs 0.4%; P = .03).[19]

Optical coherence tomography can be used to assess thrombus burden and has been shown to be more sensitive than angiographic assessment owing its high resolution.[20] In a substudy of TOTAL that prospectively enrolled 214 patients from 13 sites in which optical coherence tomography was performed immediately after thrombectomy or PCI alone and then repeated after stent deployment, there was no significant different in the pre-stent thrombus burden as a percentage of the segment analyzed among those who underwent thrombectomy compared with conventional PCI (2.36% vs 2.88%; $P = .37$).[21]

The TAPAS, TASTE, and TOTAL trials were analyzed in a pooled meta-analysis combining the 19,047 patients enrolled in all 3 studies. There was no significant difference in the incidence of 30-day cardiovascular death (2.4% vs 2.9%; $P = .06$) among those randomized to undergo manual aspiration thrombectomy compared with conventional PCI alone. There was similarly no difference in the pooled analysis with respect to recurrent myocardial infarction, stent thrombosis, heart failure, or target vessel revascularization. In a subgroup analysis of patients with high thrombus burden (defined as TIMI thrombus grade of ≥3), those treated with aspiration thrombectomy had fewer cardiovascular deaths (2.5% vs 3.1%; $P = .03$) and had more strokes or transient ischemic attacks (0.9% vs 0.5%; $P = .04$).[6]

Aspiration thrombectomy has also been investigated particularly with respect to the prevention and management of the coronary no-reflow phenomenon, which occurs when cardiac tissue fails to perfuse normally despite opening of the occluded vessel and is thought to be physiologically mediated by vessel injury related to ischemia, reperfusion, endothelial dysfunction, and distal thromboembolism. Although 1 meta-analysis of 18 studies investigating the use of aspiration thrombectomy during primary PCI versus primary PCI alone demonstrated a significant reduction in the incidence of no-reflow (relative risk, 0.63; 95% confidence interval, 0.40–0.98), there was no evidence of long-term clinical benefit with respect to all-cause mortality or target vessel or lesion revascularization.[22]

Despite initial enthusiasm for manual aspiration thrombectomy based on the results of small meta-analyses and a single-center randomized controlled trial, subsequent large, multicenter trials have demonstrated a lack of evidence supporting the routine use of thrombectomy in STEMI.

Mechanical Thrombectomy

There are very few data comparing manual and mechanical aspiration thrombectomy devices. The TREAT-MI study randomized 201 patients admitted with STEMI undergoing PCI to undergo treatment with either manual or mechanical aspiration thrombectomy before stent deployment. Manual aspiration was associated with more frequent ST-segment resolution (56.6% vs 44%; $P = .06$), but there was no difference in the primary outcome—a composite of cardiac death, recurrent MI, or target vessel revascularization at 3-year follow-up—between the 2 groups ($P = .35$).[23]

The efficacy of mechanical aspiration thrombectomy devices was further assessed in a meta-analysis of 1598 patients enrolled in 7 clinical trials demonstrated no difference between the mechanical thrombectomy and conventional PCI arms with respect to major adverse cardiac events ($P = .77$), mortality ($P = .57$), recurrent MI ($P = .32$), target vessel revascularization ($P = .19$), or final infarct size ($P = .47$). There was a trend toward a higher incidence of stroke (1.3% vs 0.4%; $P = .07$) among those treated with mechanical thrombectomy in all 7 trials evaluated.[24]

CURRENT GUIDELINES

The 2015 American College of Cardiology/ American Heart Association/Society for Cardiovascular Angiography & Intervention guidelines were updated so that routine thrombectomy during primary PCI for STEMI has been given a class III indication owing to lack of clinical benefit. Selective or bailout thrombectomy has been given a class IIb indication owing to lack of data.[25] Similarly, in the 2017 European Society of Cardiology guidelines, the use of routine aspiration thrombectomy was changed from a class IIa recommendation in 2012 to a class III recommendation.[26]

SUMMARY AND RECOMMENDATIONS

A limitation of primary PCI in STEMI is distal embolization of thrombus, which can lead to impairment of microvascular perfusion. Measures of abnormal microvascular perfusion, including angiographic blush grade and delayed ST-segment resolution, have been associated with increased mortality and worsened clinical outcomes. Large multicenter randomized controlled trials and multiple meta-analyses have failed to demonstrate an improvement in clinical outcomes with the routine use of manual aspiration thrombectomy, with some studies suggesting an increased incidence of stroke, likely owing to thrombus dislodgement during retrieval leading to cerebral vessel embolization. In patients with high thrombus burden who do not respond to balloon predilation, the use of manual aspiration thrombectomy as a bailout treatment strategy can be considered.

DISCLOSURE

The authors have no relevant disclosures regarding this article.

REFERENCES

1. Henriques JPS, Zijlstra F, Ottervanger JP, et al. Incidence and clinical significance of distal embolization during primary angioplasty for acute myocardial infarction. Eur Heart J 2002;23(14): 1112–7.

2. Sianos G, Papafaklis MI, Daemen J, et al. Angiographic stent thrombosis after routine use of drug-eluting stents in ST-segment elevation myocardial infarction: the importance of thrombus burden. J Am Coll Cardiol 2007;50(7):573–83.

3. Alak A, Jolly SS. The role of manual aspiration thrombectomy in patients undergoing primary percutaneous coronary intervention for STEMI. Curr Cardiol Rep 2016;18(3):30.

4. Stone GW, Peterson MA, Lansky AJ, et al. Impact of normalized myocardial perfusion after successful angioplasty in acute myocardial infarction. J Am Coll Cardiol 2002;39(4):591–7.

5. Ribeiro DRP, Cambruzzi E, Schmidt MM, et al. Thrombosis in ST-elevation myocardial infarction: insights from thrombi retrieved by aspiration thrombectomy. World J Cardiol 2016;8(6):362–7.

6. Jolly SS, James S, Džavík V, et al. Thrombus aspiration in ST-segment–elevation myocardial infarction. Circulation 2017;135(2):143–52.

7. Svilaas T, Vlaar PJ, van der Horst IC, et al. Thrombus aspiration during primary percutaneous coronary intervention. N Engl J Med 2008;358(6): 557–67.

8. Vlaar PJ, Svilaas T, van der Horst IC, et al. Cardiac death and reinfarction after 1 year in the thrombus aspiration during percutaneous coronary intervention in acute myocardial infarction study (TAPAS): a 1-year follow-up study. Lancet 2008;371(9628): 1915–20.

9. Kushner FG, Hand M, Smith SC, et al. 2009 focused updates: ACC/AHA guidelines for the management of patients with ST-elevation myocardial infarction (updating the 2004 guideline and 2007 focused update) and ACC/AHA/SCAI guidelines on percutaneous coronary intervention (updating the 2005 guideline and 2007 focused update): a report of the American College of Cardiology Foundation/American Heart Association Task Force on Practice Guidelines. J Am Coll Cardiol 2009;54(23):2205–41.

10. Members AF, Steg PG, James SK, et al. ESC guidelines for the management of acute myocardial infarction in patients presenting with ST-segment elevation. The Task Force on the management of ST-segment elevation acute myocardial infarction of the European Society of Cardiology (ESC). Eur Heart J 2012;33(20):2569–619.

11. Tamhane UU, Chetcuti S, Hameed I, et al. Safety and efficacy of thrombectomy in patients undergoing primary percutaneous coronary intervention for Acute ST elevation MI: a meta-analysis of randomized controlled trials. BMC Cardiovasc Disord 2010; 10(1):10.

12. Burzotta F, De Vita M, Gu YL, et al. Clinical impact of thrombectomy in acute ST-elevation myocardial infarction: an individual patient-data pooled analysis of 11 trials. Eur Heart J 2009;30(18):2193–203.

13. Bavry AA, Kumbhani DJ, Bhatt DL. Role of adjunctive thrombectomy and embolic protection devices in acute myocardial infarction: a comprehensive meta-analysis of randomized trials. Eur Heart J 2008;29(24):2989–3001.

14. Stone GW, Maehara A, Witzenbichler B, et al. Intracoronary abciximab and aspiration thrombectomy in patients with large anterior myocardial infarction: the INFUSE-AMI randomized trial. JAMA 2012; 307(17):1817–26.

15. Fröbert O, Lagerqvist B, Olivecrona GK, et al. Thrombus aspiration during ST-segment elevation myocardial infarction. N Engl J Med 2013;369(17): 1587–97.

16. Lagerqvist B, Fröbert O, Olivecrona GK, et al. Outcomes 1 year after thrombus aspiration for myocardial infarction. N Engl J Med 2014;371(12):1111–20.

17. Kumbhani DJ, Bavry AA, Desai MY, et al. Aspiration thrombectomy in patients undergoing primary angioplasty: totality of data to 2013. Catheter Cardiovasc Interv 2014;84(6):973–7.

18. Jolly SS, Cairns JA, Yusuf S, et al. Randomized trial of primary PCI with or without routine manual thrombectomy. N Engl J Med 2015;372(15):1389–98.

19. Jolly SS, Cairns JA, Lavi S, et al. Thrombus aspiration in patients with high thrombus burden in the total trial. J Am Coll Cardiol 2018;72(14):1589–96.

20. Kajander OA, Koistinen LS, Eskola M, et al. Feasibility and repeatability of optical coherence tomography measurements of pre-stent thrombus burden in patients with STEMI treated with primary PCI. Eur Heart J Cardiovasc Imaging 2015;16(1):96–107.

21. Bhindi R, Kajander OA, Jolly SS, et al. Culprit lesion thrombus burden after manual thrombectomy or percutaneous coronary intervention-alone in ST-segment elevation myocardial infarction: the optical coherence tomography sub-study of the TOTAL

(ThrOmbecTomy versus PCI ALone) trial. Eur Heart J 2015;36(29):1892–900.

22. Mancini JG, Filion KB, Windle SB, et al. Meta-analysis of the long-term effect of routine aspiration thrombectomy in patients undergoing primary percutaneous coronary intervention. Am J Cardiol 2016;118(1):23–31.

23. Vink MA, Patterson MS, van Etten J, et al. A randomized comparison of manual versus mechanical thrombus removal in primary percutaneous coronary intervention in the treatment of ST-segment elevation myocardial infarction (TREAT-MI). Catheter Cardiovasc Interv 2011;78(1): 14–9.

24. Kumbhani DJ, Bavry AA, Desai MY, et al. Role of aspiration and mechanical thrombectomy in patients with acute myocardial infarction undergoing primary angioplasty: an updated meta-analysis of randomized trials. J Am Coll Cardiol 2013;62(16): 1409–18.

25. Levine GN, Bates ER, Blankenship JC, et al. 2015 ACC/AHA/SCAI focused update on primary percutaneous coronary intervention for patients with ST-elevation myocardial infarction: an update of the 2011 ACCF/AHA/SCAI guideline for percutaneous coronary intervention and the 2013 ACCF/AHA guideline for the management of ST-elevation myocardial infarction. J Am Coll Cardiol 2016; 67(10):1235–50.

26. Ibanez B, James S, Agewall S, et al. 2017 ESC guidelines for the management of acute myocardial infarction in patients presenting with ST-segment elevation: the task force for the management of acute myocardial infarction in patients presenting with ST-segment elevation of the European Society of Cardiology (ESC). Eur Heart J 2018;39(2): 119–77.

Optical Coherence Tomography in Acute Coronary Syndromes

Keyvan Karimi Galougahi, MD, PhD[a,b,c],
Evan Shlofmitz, DO[d], Allen Jeremias, MD, MSc[d],
Gregory Petrossian, BS[d], Gary S. Mintz, MD[e],
Akiko Maehara, MD[d,e,f], Richard Shlofmitz, MD[d],
Ziad A. Ali, MD, DPhil[d,e,f],*

KEYWORDS

- Myocardial infarction • Acute coronary syndromes • Optical coherence tomography
- Intravascular ultrasound • Percutaneous coronary intervention

KEY POINTS

- Intravascular optical coherence tomography enables assessment of the culprit plaque morphology in ACS.
- Atherothrombotic substrates for ACS consist of plaque rupture, erosion, and calcified nodule.
- Optical coherence tomography allows for effective treatment of patients presenting with ACS by PCI.

INTRODUCTION

Major insights into the pathobiology of coronary atherosclerosis have originally been gained from post mortem histopathologic studies.[1–3] Advances in intravascular imaging technology, especially optical coherence tomography (OCT), have enabled an in-depth understanding of the major triggers and substrates for atherothrombotic events that lead to acute coronary syndromes (ACS). In this review, we provide a summary of intracoronary OCT data on the atherothrombotic (plaque rupture, plaque erosion, and calcific nodules) and the rarer nonatherothrombotic causes of ACS (spontaneous coronary artery dissection [SCAD], coronary artery spasm, and coronary embolism). We discuss the usefulness of intravascular imaging for effective treatment of patients presenting with ACS by transcatheter and medical therapies.

ATHEROTHROMBOTIC CULPRIT LESIONS ASSESSED BY INTRAVASCULAR IMAGING

A detailed in vivo characterization of coronary plaque morphology in ACS is feasible by using intravascular imaging modalities, such as intravascular ultrasound (IVUS) examination[4] and OCT.[5] During OCT acquisition, the near-infrared light spectrum is directed at the vessel wall while the blood is flushed from the coronary artery lumen. OCT generates high-resolution, cross-sectional, and 3-dimensional images of the vessel. Overall, OCT light has lower penetration depth than the ultrasound waves in IVUS examination, which limits OCT imaging, particularly in the presence of highly attenuating structures such as red thrombus or lipid and necrotic core.[6] OCT generates images with greater axial resolution compared with IVUS examination (Fig. 1).

[a] Royal Prince Alfred Hospital, Sydney, Australia; [b] University of Sydney, Sydney, Australia; [c] Heart Research Institute, 7 Eliza Street, Newtown, NSW 2042, Australia; [d] The Heart Center, St Francis Hospital, 100 Port Washington Blvd, Flower Hill, NY 11576, USA; [e] Cardiovascular Research Foundation, 1700 Broadway, 9th Floor, New York, NY 10019, USA; [f] New York-Presbyterian Hospital/Columbia University Irving Medical Center, New York, NY, USA
* Corresponding author. Heart Research Institute, 7 Eliza Street, Newtown, NSW 2042, Australia
E-mail address: ziad.ali@dcvi.org

Intervent Cardiol Clin 10 (2021) 323–332
https://doi.org/10.1016/j.iccl.2021.03.004
2211-7458/21/© 2021 Elsevier Inc. All rights reserved.

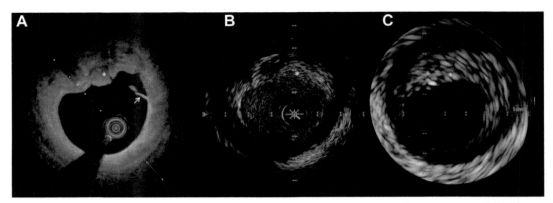

Fig. 1. Intravascular imaging of plaque rupture in a patient with non–ST-segment elevation myocardial infarction. (A) OCT of a ruptured cap (arrow) overlying the typical hollow crater appearance associated with mixed thrombus (asterisk). (B) On high-definition (60 MHz) IVUS examination, the disrupted cap is not as clearly defined as OCT, and thrombus (asterisk) is less clearly delineated. Depth penetration is limited owing to the presence of lipidic plaque. (C) IVUS examination at 20 MHz does not allow visualization of plaque rupture or the thrombus. Depth penetration is superior.

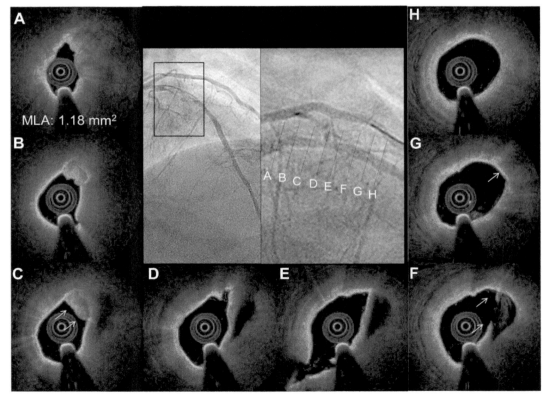

Fig. 2. ST-segment elevation myocardial infarction with RFC (plaque rupture). Angiography in a patient presenting with ST-segment elevation myocardial infarction showed stenosis in the left anterior descending coronary artery (inset). Serial optical coherence tomographic cross-sectional imaging with co-registration from proximal to distal of the culprit lesion following aspiration thrombectomy identified (A) the minimal luminal area (MLA) in an area of necrotic core, (B, C) adherent white thrombus (arrow), (D, E) empty crater from plaque rupture, (F) thin-cap fibroatheroma (TCFA) rupture (arrows), (G) intact TCFA (arrow), and (H) lipidic plaque. (Adapted from Ali ZA, Karimi Galougahi K, Maehara A, et al. Intracoronary optical coherence tomography 2018: current status and future directions. JACC Cardiovasc Interv. 2017;10(24):2473-2487[6] with permission from Elsevier.)

On OCT imaging in ACS, culprit lesions are broadly categorized into plaques with ruptured fibrous cap (RFC) or with intact fibrous caps (IFC),[7] which correlate with the histopathologic classification of plaque rupture and plaque erosion, respectively.[7] On OCT imaging, plaques with RFC are characterized with thrombi in association with discontinuity in a thin fibrous cap that overlies a cavity or lipid-rich core (Fig. 2).[5,8] OCT-defined "definite" culprit plaques with IFC are characterized as the presence of a luminal thrombus overlying an intact and visualized plaque (Fig. 3), whereas "probable" OCT-defined culprit plaques with IFC are defined as (1) luminal surface irregularity at the culprit lesion in the absence of thrombus or (2) the attenuation of the underlying plaque by a thrombus without a superficial lipid or calcification immediately proximal or distal to the site of the thrombus.[5,8] Eruptive calcified nodules

are defined as the expulsion of small calcific nodules into the lumen.[9] In OCT studies, plaque rupture is responsible for 50% of ACS, whereas plaque erosion, calcified nodule, SCAD, and other causes constitute the underlying etiologies in 37%, 3%, 2%, and 8% of the cases, respectively.[6]

Culprit Plaque with Ruptured Fibrous Cap (Plaque Rupture) on Optical Coherence Tomography

ACS secondary to plaques with RFC portends worse prognosis compared with ACS owing to plaques with IFC.[10,11] A thin-cap fibroatheroma (TCFA) is the most likely lesion precursor for ACS owing to ruptured plaques.[5,12–15] TCFAs tend to cluster in the proximal segment of the left anterior descending artery, whereas 2 clustering sites in the right coronary artery and 1 clustering site in the circumflex artery are

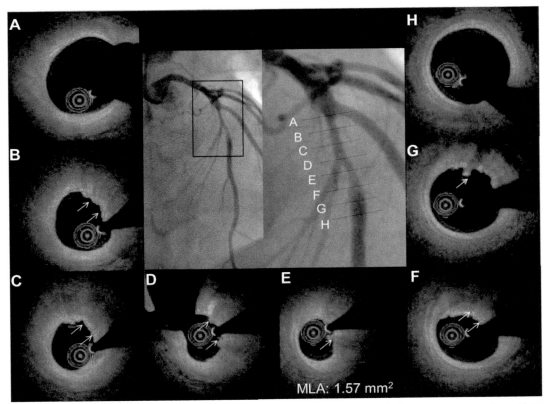

MLA: 1.57 mm²

Fig. 3. ST-segment elevation myocardial infarction with IFC (erosion). Angiography in a patient presenting with ST-segment elevation myocardial infarction showed stenosis in the left anterior descending coronary artery (*inset*). Serial optical coherence tomographic cross-sectional imaging with co-registration from proximal to distal of the culprit lesion (*A–H*) identified thrombus (mostly white thrombus, *arrows*) without RFC, indicating plaque erosion. (*Adapted from* Ali ZA, Karimi Galougahi K, Maehara A, et al. Intracoronary optical coherence tomography 2018: current status and future directions. *JACC Cardiovasc Interv.* 2017;10(24):2473-2487[6] with permission from Elsevier.)

observed on 3-vessel OCT in patients with ACS.[16] In contrast, no obvious patterns are discerned in the distribution of TCFAs in patients without ACS.[16,17]

Although TCFAs are considered the likely lesion precursors for RFC, the risk of acute myocardial infarction (MI) or sudden cardiac death related to TCFAs is low as observed in the Providing Regional Observations to Study Predictors of Events in the Coronary Tree (PROSPECT) trial and other imaging studies.[18,19] These findings are consistent with pathologic studies demonstrating that many plaques destabilize without resulting in a clinical syndrome.[20] A thrombus associated with plaque rupture or erosion may be contained with the process of healing; nonetheless, in specific occasions, a prothrombotic milieu may coincide with plaque rupture and culminate in ACS.[21] Based on these observations, healed plaque ruptures or erosions may be considered a signature of an aborted ACS. The characteristics of healed coronary plaques on OCT include heterogeneous signal-rich layers of different optical densities.[22,23]

The ability of OCT to determine the site of plaque rupture, thrombus burden, and the longitudinal extent of underlying plaque, as well as to accurately measure reference lumen and vessel diameters, suggests the usefulness of OCT to guide primary PCI in ACS. By OCT assessment in TROFI (Randomized study to Assess the Effect of Thrombus Aspiration on Flow Area in Patients With STEMI), in 141 patients with ST-segment elevation MI (STEMI), manual thrombectomy did not increase the effective flow area or minimal stent area.[24] Although routine aspiration thrombectomy in STEMI is not recommended, a retrospective OCT-based study reported a correlation between the post-thrombectomy residual thrombus and the extent of microvascular dysfunction and myocardial damage, suggesting a potential use of thrombectomy in lesions with a high thrombus burden to decrease distal embolization and preserve microcirculatory function.[14] This approach requires prospective validation before adoption in clinical practice.

In a retrospective analysis of 588 lesions in 507 patients in CLI-OPCI ACS (Centro per la Lotta Contro L'Infarto-Optimization of Percutaneous Coronary Intervention Database Undergoing PCI for ACS), predictors of stent-related events on OCT were similar to the elective setting: underexpansion (minimal stent area <4.5 mm² [hazard ratio (HR), 2.72; $P < .01$), stent inflow/outflow disease (reference luminal area <4.5 mm² at the distal [HR, 6.07; $P < .001$] or

proximal [HR, 8.50; $P < .001$] stent edges), and dissection at the distal stent edge of greater than 200 μm (HR, 3.84; $P < .001$).[25] Additionally, intrastent plaque or thrombus protrusion (HR, 2.35; $P < .01$) was an independent predictor of adverse outcomes.[25]

In a 2:1 propensity-matched prospective cohort study, prestenting and poststenting OCT guidance in 214 patients with STEMI resulted in larger final minimum lumen diameter compared with angiographic guidance in 428 patients (2.99 ± 0.48 mm vs 2.79 ± 0.47 mm; $P < .0001$), potentially because of further postdilatation in suboptimally deployed stents in the OCT arm.[26] In the randomized DOCTORS study (Does Optical Coherence Tomography Optimize Results of Stenting), higher post-PCI fractional flow reserve values were achieved with OCT guidance versus angiography guidance in 240 patients with non-STEMI (0.94 ± 0.04 vs 0.92 ± 0.05; $P < .005$).[27] Appropriately powered randomized controlled trials are warranted to substantiate the potential benefits for the OCT-guided optimization of PCI in STEMI that are suggested by the nonrandomized studies.

Culprit Plaque with Intact Fibrous Caps (Erosion) on Optical Coherence Tomography

Compared with plaques with RFC (see Fig. 2), plaques with IFC (see Fig. 3) have less severe diameter stenosis (64.4 ± 13.3% vs 68.6 ± 13.8%; $P < .001$), minimal lumen area (1.8 mm² [1.4–2.8 mm²] vs 1.6 mm² [1.3–2.2 mm²]; $P = .001$),[28] a lower lipid content, a thicker fibrous caps, smaller lipid arcs, less calcification,[28–30] and more often occur near bifurcations[28,29] in younger patients, especially women, without traditional cardiovascular risk factors, except for smoking.[28] The proximity of the plaques with IFC to bifurcations may suggest a role for alterations in flow and shear stress near bifurcations in the pathogenesis of erosions. Alterations in laminar flow result in the activation of innate immunity with neutrophil recruitment,[31] and activation of adaptive immunity with CD8+ T-lymphocyte recruitment and adhesion,[29] eventually leading to endothelial damage and thrombus formation.

TCFAs are less frequently observed in erosions than in ruptures (14% vs 90%; $P < .001$). More erosions occur in the left anterior descending artery as compared with ruptures (61% vs 47%), whereas the opposite is true in the right coronary artery (31% vs 43%), and lesions are observed with similar frequency in the left circumflex artery (8% vs 10%; $P = .002$).[29] Both erosions and ruptures occur more frequently in the proximal and mid segments of coronary arteries. Multivessel disease is more common in ruptures than in erosions (50% vs 30%; $P < .001$).[29] In ACS secondary to plaque erosion, more lipidic plaques (53.9% vs 41.8%; $P = .039$), macrophage accumulation (59.8% vs 41.8%; $P = .002$), and calcification (34.2% vs 21.8%; $P = .020$) are noted on OCT in patients presenting with initial Thrombolysis In Myocardial Infarction (TIMI) flow of 1 or less compared with patients with higher initial TIMI flow grades.[32]

In a single-center, nonrandomized, uncontrolled study of patients with ACS secondary to OCT-defined erosion (n = 55), patients with a residual diameter stenosis of less than 70% on coronary angiography (after manual thrombectomy in 46 patients [83.6%]) were treated with antithrombotic therapy without stenting (glycoprotein IIb/IIIa inhibitor in 35 [63.6%] plus aspirin and ticagrelor in all patients).[33] Among 53 patients who completed the 12-month follow-up, 49 (92.5%) remained free from major adverse cardiovascular events; 3 patients (5.7%) required revascularization because of exertional angina and 1 patient (1.9%) had gastrointestinal bleeding.[34] Among 52 patients who completed a median follow-up of 4.8 years, there were no incidences of death, MIs, strokes, bypass surgeries, or heart failure, although 11 patients (21.1%) underwent elective target lesion revascularization.[35] The patients who did not require target lesion revascularization during the follow-up had a greater decrease in thrombus volume on repeat OCT at 1 month compared with the group who required revascularization (95% vs 45%; $P = .001$).[35] Large randomized controlled trials are warranted to establish whether a no-stenting approach is safe and effective in ACS secondary to plaque erosions.

Calcified Nodule on Optical Coherence Tomography

Three types of calcified plaques are identified on OCT at the culprit lesion sites in ACS: an eruptive calcified nodule, a superficial calcific sheet, and a calcified protrusion.[9] A superficial calcific sheet, also called sheet calcium in histopathology, is defined as a sheet-like superficial calcific plate without erupted nodules or a mass protruding into the lumen, minimal or no visible disruption of overlying fibrous tissue, and minimal compromise of the lumen. A calcified protrusion, also called protruding nodular calcification in histopathology, is defined as a protruding calcific mass with a smooth leading edge, without eruptive nodules that are the hallmark of eruptive calcified nodules.[9]

Eruptive calcified nodules identified in the nonculprit segments of the left anterior descending artery portend worse prognosis compared with calcified protrusions (death and MI rate of 20% vs 3.3% at 1 year; $P < .001$).[36] On OCT, calcified nodules were present in 6% of patients undergoing PCI in a single center study, either in patients with stable coronary disease or in culprit lesions of ACS.[37] In culprit lesions, superficial calcific sheet is the most common type (67.4%), followed by eruptive calcified nodule (25.5%) and calcified protrusion (7.1%). The role of calcific sheets and calcified protrusions in causing ACS is not known. It is likely that these plaque types are "bystanders" at the culprit lesion site; nevertheless, more studies are needed to clarify their putative role in ACS. Consistent with histopathologic reports, eruptive calcified nodules are frequently located in the mid right coronary artery where cyclic hinge movement may cause a weakening of calcified plaques leading to fracture.[9,38] A superficial calcific sheet is most frequently found in the left anterior descending artery.[9] Red thrombus is predominant in eruptive calcified nodules and white thrombus is predominant in superficial calcific sheets.[9]

The treatment of calcific plaques in ACS is challenging (Fig. 4). The minimal stent area is the smallest area in a primary PCI on the calcified nodule compared with erosion and plaque rupture.[39] Stent edge dissection and stent malapposition are frequently observed in PCI on eruptive calcified nodules compared with superficial calcific sheet and calcified protrusion, whereas the minimal stent area is smallest after intervention on a superficial calcific sheet among the 3 calcific lesion subtypes.[40] A superficial calcific sheet and calcified nodules and protrusions may, therefore, need modification with rotational or orbital atherectomy to avoid suboptimal PCI results (see Fig. 4), nonetheless the use of these devices is contraindicated in thrombotic lesions.

NONATHEROTHROMBOTIC CAUSES OF ACUTE CORONARY SYNDROMES ASSESSED BY INTRAVASCULAR IMAGING

Intravascular imaging, particularly OCT, can be useful in diagnosing the infrequent causes of ACS and guiding their management.

Spontaneous Coronary Artery Dissection on Optical Coherence Tomography

On angiography, SCAD may appear as contrast staining in the arterial wall associated with multiple radiolucent lumens (type 1), diffuse stenosis

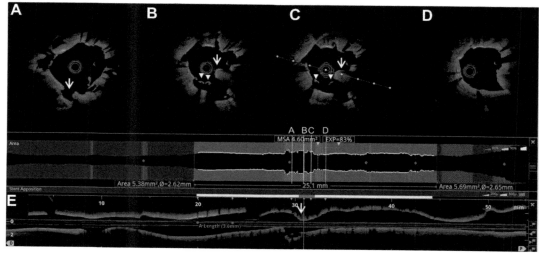

Fig. 4. The impact of calcific protrusion on percutaneous coronary intervention. On post-percutaneous coronary intervention (PCI) OCT imaging in a patient with ACS, in whom pre-PCI OCT imaging was not performed, calcified protrusion is visualized, which was identified as thrombus by the operator on angiography. On OCT imaging (A) tissue disruption (arrow), (B, C) penetration of the nodular calcification through the stent struts (arrow) with associated severe malapposition (arrowheads), (D) and minimal disease proximally are noted, (E) Position of the protruding nodule is identified on the longitudinal pullback (arrow).

of varying length and severity with abrupt change in the arterial caliber from the normal diameter to diffuse narrowing (type 2, most common appearance, usually >20 mm), or focal or tubular stenosis mimicking atherosclerosis (type 3, usually <20 mm).[41] SCAD is often asymptomatic, but it can infrequently be the underlying cause of ACS. SCAD mainly affects women (>90% of cases), most commonly those between 44 and 55 years of age.[42] SCAD can propagate in antero-grade or retrograde directions, and the mean length of dissection is typically greater than 45 mm on quantitative coronary angiography.[43] Thus, the tear may not be located at the proximal edge of the intramural hematoma (Fig. 5) and often it is remote from the proximal edge of the hematoma as the blood can traverse through the low resistance dissection planes owing to the absence of atherosclerosis.

A diagnosis of type 2 or type 3 SCAD often requires intravascular imaging after the administration of intracoronary vasodilators to exclude vasospasm, which visualize an intramural hematoma or true and false lumens. OCT provides visualization of intimal tears, intraluminal thrombi, false lumen, and intramural hematoma (see Fig. 5); however, owing to limited penetration depth, OCT may not delineate the entire thickness of the intramural hematoma.[44] It is critical to note the potential risks associated with intracoronary imaging in SCAD, including the potential to extend the dissection with the guide

wire or imaging catheter, guide catheter-induced iatrogenic dissection, hydraulic extension by contrast injection required in OCT, and imaging catheter-induced coronary occlusion.[41] Therefore, intracoronary imaging in suspected SCAD should only be performed if required for diagnosis or to guide treatment, using meticulous techniques. In this regard, IVUS examination may be the preferred modality for safety.

Conservative medical therapy and lifestyle modifications are the mainstays of management in SCAD, with revascularization by PCI or bypass grafting reserved for unstable patients. Intravascular imaging can confirm the true lumen before stent implantation and optimization of stent deployment. Long stents (5–10 mm longer on both edges of the intramural hematoma) are typically needed to ensure the prevention of hematoma propagation caused by compression during stent deployment.[41] For longer lesions that require multiple stents, a multistep approach starting by stenting the distal edge, followed by the proximal edge, and finishing by stenting the middle segment may be useful in preventing extension of the intramural hematoma.[45]

Coronary Artery Spasm on Optical Coherence Tomography
Coronary artery spasm is defined as a more than 90% decrease in the luminal diameter with myocardial ischemia that is relieved by

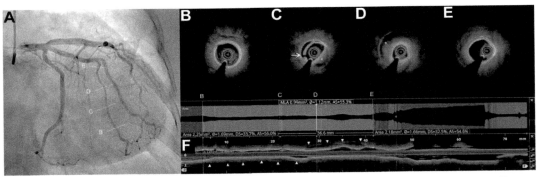

Fig. 5. ACS caused by SCAD. (*A*) Angiography in a middle-aged woman presenting with ACS revealed diffuse stenosis with an abrupt change in the arterial caliber in a branch of the ramus intermedius. The demographics, absence of atherosclerotic plaques in the remainder of vessels, and the angiographic appearance were highly suggestive of SCAD. OCT imaging performed after administration of intracoronary nitroglycerine shows the (*B*) distal normal vessel, (*C*) site of intimal disruption (*arrow*), (*D*) minimal lumen area owing to compression from an intramural hematoma (*asterisk*), and (*E*) proximal normal reference segment. (*F*) Longitudinal imaging shows the extent of intramural hematoma (*arrowheads*).

vasodilators.[46] The prevalence of coronary spasm varies depending on the population studied and whether physiologic measures (fractional flow reserve, coronary flow reserve, and index of microvascular resistance) and provocative testing with ergonovine or acetylcholine are performed.[47,48] Coronary vasospasm can occur in patients with or without atherosclerosis.[48]

Because a significant proportion of patients with coronary spasm present with ACS, coronary artery spasm should be included in the differential diagnosis of patients presenting with MI and nonobstructive coronary arteries.[47,48] On OCT, coronary spasm may be evident as intimal bumping.[49] Plaque erosion at the site of coronary spasm is common, and spasm tends to be more pronounced at branch points and nonplaque sites.[50] These findings indicate that vasospastic sites are rarely normal and that plaque erosion with thrombus is a frequent finding, suggesting a role for antiplatelet therapy in combination with vasodilators.

Coronary Artery Embolism on Optical Coherence Tomography

Several conditions predispose to coronary embolism as a cause of ACS, including thrombophilia, atrial fibrillation, valvular disease, patent foramen ovale, infective endocarditis, and nonbacterial thrombotic endocarditis.[51] Angiography together with a high index of suspicion in patients with risk factors are pivotal in the diagnosis of coronary embolism. Angiographic features, including heavy thrombus burden, abrupt occlusion, or involvement of multiple coronary territories can provide clues to an embolic

phenomenon. The unaffected coronary vessels might seem to be normal without significant atherosclerotic disease, and the lack of collaterals to the occluded territory might suggest embolism. The absence of a plaque rupture or erosion on OCT after thrombectomy aids in diagnosing coronary embolus.[52] Thromboembolism can also occur in the acute phase of ACS from plaque rupture to the downstream coronary territory.[53,54] Additional imaging modalities might be necessary for further assessment, such as transesophageal echocardiography, to evaluate the left atrial appendage or transthoracic echocardiography with a bubble study to identify atrial shunts,[53,55] and determine the appropriate management.

SUMMARY

Mechanistic insights gained by histopathologic studies have subsequently been reproduced in vivo by intravascular imaging, especially by high-resolution OCT imaging. Although culprit lesions in more than one-half of the patients presenting with ACS are plaques with ruptured caps, plaque erosions are responsible for ACS in more than one-third of cases. A conservative no-stenting approach with antithrombotic therapy is supported in small, nonrandomized studies and warrants testing in large, randomized trials. Intracoronary OCT is also a useful adjunctive tool in the diagnosis and appropriate management of the rare causes of ACS, such as eruptive calcified nodules, SCAD, and coronary spasm or embolism. The existing data that support the use of intravascular OCT to optimize primary PCI and improve long-term outcomes in ACS warrant testing in statistically powered randomized controlled trials.

CLINICS CARE POINTS

- On OCT, culprit lesions for ACS are categorized into plaques with ruptured fibrous cap or with intact fibrous cap, which correlate with the histopathologic classification of plaque rupture and plaque erosion, respectively.
- By OCT assessment, plaque rupture is responsible for 50% and plaque erosion for 37% of patients with ACS.
- Eruptive calcified nodules are rarer causes of ACS, responsible for 3% of all cases by OCT assessment.

DISCLOSURE

K. Karimi Galougahi: None. E. Shlofmitz: Consultant - Abbott Vascular, Medtronic, Opsens Medical. A. Jeremias: Institutional funding (unrestricted education grant) and serves as a consultant for Volcano/Philips and Abbott Vascular; consultant to ACIST Medical and Boston Scientific. G. Petrossian: None. G.S. Mintz: Honoraria - Abiomed, Boston Scientific, Medtronic, and Philips. A. Maehara: Grant support and consultant - Abbott Vascular and Boston Scientific. R. Shlofmitz: Speaker – Shockwave. Z.A. Ali: Institutional research grants to Columbia University – Abbott, Cardiovascular Systems Inc; consultant – Amgen, AstraZeneca, Boston Scientific; equity – Shockwave.

REFERENCES

1. Burke AP, Farb A, Malcom GT, et al. Coronary risk factors and plaque morphology in men with coronary disease who died suddenly. N Engl J Med 1997;336(18):1276–82.
2. Farb A, Tang AL, Burke AP, et al. Sudden coronary death. Frequency of active coronary lesions, inactive coronary lesions, and myocardial infarction. Circulation 1995;92(7):1701–9.
3. Virmani R, Kolodgie FD, Burke AP, et al. Lessons from sudden coronary death: a comprehensive morphological classification scheme for atherosclerotic lesions. Arterioscler Thromb Vasc Biol 2000; 20(5):1262–75.
4. Kotani J, Mintz GS, Castagna MT, et al. Intravascular ultrasound analysis of infarct-related and non-infarct-related arteries in patients who presented with an acute myocardial infarction. Circulation 2003;107(23):2889–93.
5. Jia H, Abtahian F, Aguirre AD, et al. In vivo diagnosis of plaque erosion and calcified nodule in patients with acute coronary syndrome by intravascular optical coherence tomography. J Am Coll Cardiol 2013;62(19):1748–58.
6. Ali ZA, Karimi Galougahi K, Maehara A, et al. Intracoronary optical coherence tomography 2018: current status and future directions. JACC Cardiovasc Interv 2017;10(24):2473–87.
7. Ozaki Y, Tanaka A, Tanimoto T, et al. Thin-cap fibroatheroma as high-risk plaque for microvascular obstruction in patients with acute coronary syndrome. Circ Cardiovasc Imaging 2011;4(6):620–7.
8. Johnson TW, Raber L, di Mario C, et al. Clinical use of intracoronary imaging. Part 2: acute coronary syndromes, ambiguous coronary angiography findings, and guiding interventional decision-making: an expert consensus document of the European Association of Percutaneous Cardiovascular Interventions. Eur Heart J 2019;40(31):2566–84.
9. Sugiyama T, Yamamoto E, Fracassi F, et al. Calcified Plaques in patients with acute coronary syndromes. JACC Cardiovasc Interv 2019;12(6):531–40.
10. Niccoli G, Montone RA, Di Vito L, et al. Plaque rupture and intact fibrous cap assessed by optical coherence tomography portend different outcomes in patients with acute coronary syndrome. Eur Heart J 2015;36(22):1377–84.
11. Hoshino M, Yonetsu T, Usui E, et al. Clinical significance of the presence or absence of lipid-rich plaque underneath intact fibrous cap plaque in acute coronary syndrome. J Am Heart Assoc 2019;8(9): e011820.
12. Guagliumi G, Capodanno D, Saia F, et al. Mechanisms of atherothrombosis and vascular response to primary percutaneous coronary intervention in women versus men with acute myocardial infarction: results of the OCTAVIA study. JACC Cardiovasc Interv 2014;7(9):958–68.
13. Wang L, Parodi G, Maehara A, et al. Variable underlying morphology of culprit plaques associated with ST-elevation myocardial infarction: an optical coherence tomography analysis from the SMART trial. Eur Heart J Cardiovasc Imaging 2015;16(12): 1381–9.
14. Higuma T, Soeda T, Abe N, et al. A combined optical coherence tomography and intravascular ultrasound study on plaque rupture, plaque erosion, and calcified nodule in patients with ST-segment elevation myocardial infarction: incidence, morphologic characteristics, and outcomes after percutaneous coronary intervention. JACC Cardiovasc Interv 2015;8(9):1166–76.
15. Kajander OA, Pinilla-Echeverri N, Jolly SS, et al. Culprit plaque morphology in STEMI - an optical coherence tomography study: insights from the

TOTAL-OCT substudy. EuroIntervention 2016;12(6): 716–23.

16. Araki M, Soeda T, Kim HO, et al. Spatial distribution of vulnerable plaques: comprehensive in vivo coronary plaque mapping. JACC Cardiovasc Imaging 2020;13(9):1989–99.

17. Pinilla-Echeverri N, Mehta SR, Wang J, et al. Nonculprit lesion plaque morphology in patients with ST-segment-elevation myocardial infarction: results from the COMPLETE trial optical coherence tomography substudys. Circ Cardiovasc Interv 2020; 13(7):e008768.

18. Stone GW, Maehara A, Lansky AJ, et al. A prospective natural-history study of coronary atherosclerosis. N Engl J Med 2011;364(3):226–35.

19. Ferencik M, Mayrhofer T, Bittner DO, et al. Use of high-risk coronary atherosclerotic plaque detection for risk stratification of patients with stable chest pain: a secondary analysis of the PROMISE randomized clinical trial. JAMA Cardiol 2018;3(2):144–52.

20. Burke AP, Kolodgie FD, Farb A, et al. Healed plaque ruptures and sudden coronary death: evidence that subclinical rupture has a role in plaque progression. Circulation 2001;103(7):934–40.

21. Arbab-Zadeh A, Fuster V. The myth of the "vulnerable plaque": transitioning from a focus on individual lesions to atherosclerotic disease burden for coronary artery disease risk assessment. J Am Coll Cardiol 2015;65(8):846–55.

22. Shimokado A, Matsuo Y, Kubo T, et al. In vivo optical coherence tomography imaging and histopathology of healed coronary plaques. Atherosclerosis 2018;275:35–42.

23. Dai J, Fang C, Zhang S, et al. Frequency, predictors, distribution, and morphological characteristics of layered culprit and nonculprit plaques of patients with acute myocardial infarction: in vivo 3-vessel optical coherence tomography study. Circ Cardiovasc Interv 2020;13(10):e009125.

24. Sabate M, Windecker S, Iniguez A, et al. Everolimus-eluting bioresorbable stent vs. durable polymer everolimus-eluting metallic stent in patients with ST-segment elevation myocardial infarction: results of the randomized ABSORB ST-segment elevation myocardial infarction-TROFI II trial. Eur Heart J 2016;37(3):229–40.

25. Prati F, Romagnoli E, Gatto L, et al. Clinical impact of suboptimal stenting and residual intrastent plaque/thrombus protrusion in patients with acute coronary syndrome: the CLI-OPCI ACS Substudy (Centro per la Lotta Contro L'Infarto-Optimization of Percutaneous Coronary Intervention in Acute Coronary Syndrome). Circ Cardiovasc Interv 2016; 9(12):e003726.

26. Sheth TN, Kajander OA, Lavi S, et al. Optical coherence tomography-guided percutaneous coronary intervention in ST-segment-elevation myocardial infarction: a prospective propensity-matched cohort of the thrombectomy versus percutaneous coronary intervention alone trial. Circ Cardiovasc Interv 2016;9(4):e003414.

27. Meneveau N, Ecarnot F, Souteyrand G, et al. Does optical coherence tomography optimize results of stenting? Rationale and study design. Am Heart J 2014;168(2):175–81. e171-172.

28. Dai J, Xing L, Jia H, et al. In vivo predictors of plaque erosion in patients with ST-segment elevation myocardial infarction: a clinical, angiographical, and intravascular optical coherence tomography study. Eur Heart J 2018;39(22): 2077–85.

29. Leistner DM, Krankel N, Meteva D, et al. Differential immunological signature at the culprit site distinguishes acute coronary syndrome with intact from acute coronary syndrome with ruptured fibrous cap: results from the prospective translational OPTICO-ACS study. Eur Heart J 2020; 41(37):3549–60.

30. Fang C, Dai J, Zhang S, et al. Culprit lesion morphology in young patients with ST-segment elevated myocardial infarction: a clinical, angiographic and optical coherence tomography study. Atherosclerosis 2019;289:94–100.

31. Franck G, Mawson T, Sausen G, et al. Flow perturbation mediates neutrophil recruitment and potentiates endothelial injury via TLR2 in mice: implications for superficial erosion. Circ Res 2017; 121(1):31–42.

32. Wang J, Fang C, Zhang S, et al. Systemic and local factors associated with reduced thrombolysis in myocardial infarction flow in ST-segment elevation myocardial infarction patients with plaque erosion detected by intravascular optical coherence tomography. Int J Cardiovasc Imaging 2021;37(2):399–409.

33. Jia H, Dai J, Hou J, et al. Effective anti-thrombotic therapy without stenting: intravascular optical coherence tomography-based management in plaque erosion (the EROSION study). Eur Heart J 2017;38(11):792–800.

34. Xing L, Yamamoto E, Sugiyama T, et al. EROSION Study (Effective anti-thrombotic therapy without stenting: intravascular optical coherence tomography-based management in plaque erosion): a 1-year follow-up report. Circ Cardiovasc Interv 2017;10(12):e005860.

35. He L, Qin Y, Xu Y, et al. Predictors of non-stenting strategy for acute coronary syndrome caused by plaque erosion: 4-year outcomes of the EROSION study. EuroIntervention 2020 [Epub ahead of print].

36. Prati F, Gatto L, Fabbiocchi F, et al. Clinical outcomes of calcified nodules detected by optical coherence tomography: a sub-analysis of the CLIMA study. EuroIntervention 2020;16(5):380–6.

37. Yamamoto MH, Maehara A, Song L, et al. Optical coherence tomography assessment of morphological characteristics in suspected coronary artery disease, but angiographically nonobstructive lesions. Cardiovasc Revasc Med 2019;20(6):475–9.

38. Lee T, Mintz GS, Matsumura M, et al. Prevalence, predictors, and clinical presentation of a calcified nodule as assessed by optical coherence tomography. JACC Cardiovasc Imaging 2017;10(8):883–91.

39. Khalifa AKM, Kubo T, Ino Y, et al. Optical coherence tomography comparison of percutaneous coronary intervention among plaque rupture, erosion, and calcified nodule in acute myocardial infarction. Circ J 2020;84(6):911–6.

40. Nakajima A, Araki M, Kurihara O, et al. Comparison of post-stent optical coherence tomography findings among three subtypes of calcified culprit plaques in patients with acute coronary syndrome. Catheter Cardiovasc Interv 2021;97(4):634–45.

41. Saw J, Mancini GBJ, Humphries KH. Contemporary review on spontaneous coronary artery dissection. J Am Coll Cardiol 2016;68(3):297–312.

42. Rogowski S, Maeder MT, Weilenmann D, et al. Spontaneous coronary artery dissection: angiographic follow-up and long-term clinical outcome in a predominantly medically treated population. Catheter Cardiovasc Interv 2017;89(1):59–68.

43. Saw J, Mancini GB, Humphries K, et al. Angiographic appearance of spontaneous coronary artery dissection with intramural hematoma proven on intracoronary imaging. Catheter Cardiovasc Interv 2016;87(2):E54–61.

44. Alfonso F, Paulo M, Gonzalo N, et al. Diagnosis of spontaneous coronary artery dissection by optical coherence tomography. J Am Coll Cardiol 2012;59(12):1073–9.

45. Walsh SJ, Jokhi PP, Saw J. Successful percutaneous management of coronary dissection and extensive intramural haematoma associated with ST elevation MI. Acute Card Care 2008;10(4):231–3.

46. Beltrame JF, Sasayama S, Maseri A. Racial heterogeneity in coronary artery vasomotor reactivity: differences between Japanese and Caucasian patients. J Am Coll Cardiol 1999;33(6):1442–52.

47. Ong P, Athanasiadis A, Hill S, et al. Coronary artery spasm as a frequent cause of acute coronary syndrome: the CASPAR (Coronary Artery Spasm in Patients With Acute Coronary Syndrome) Study. J Am Coll Cardiol 2008;52(7):523–7.

48. Nakayama N, Kaikita K, Fukunaga T, et al. Clinical features and prognosis of patients with coronary spasm-induced non-ST-segment elevation acute coronary syndrome. J Am Heart Assoc 2014;3(3):e000795.

49. Reynolds HR, Maehara A, Kwong RY, et al. Coronary optical coherence tomography and cardiac magnetic resonance imaging to determine underlying causes of MINOCA in Women. Circulation 2021;143(7):624–40.

50. Nakagawa H, Morikawa Y, Mizuno Y, et al. Coronary spasm preferentially occurs at branch points: an angiographic comparison with atherosclerotic plaque. Circ Cardiovasc Interv 2009;2(2):97–104.

51. Waterbury TM, Tarantini G, Vogel B, et al. Non-atherosclerotic causes of acute coronary syndromes. Nat Rev Cardiol 2020;17(4):229–41.

52. Soverow J, Hastings R, Ali Z. OCT-guided management of a pregnant woman with ST-elevation myocardial infarction. Int J Cardiol 2016;215:135–7.

53. Raphael CE, Heit JA, Reeder GS, et al. Coronary embolus: an underappreciated cause of acute coronary syndromes. JACC Cardiovasc Interv 2018;11(2):172–80.

54. Takahata M, Ino Y, Kubo T, et al. Prevalence, features, and prognosis of artery-to-artery embolic ST-segment-elevation myocardial infarction: an optical coherence tomography study. J Am Heart Assoc 2020;9(24):e017661.

55. Shibata T, Kawakami S, Noguchi T, et al. Prevalence, clinical features, and prognosis of acute myocardial infarction attributable to coronary artery embolism. Circulation 2015;132(4):241–50.

Management of Multivessel Disease and Physiology Testing in ST Elevation Myocardial Infarction

Shanthosh Sivapathan, MBBS, MPH[a],
Prajith Jeyaprakash, BMed, MD, MMed[a],
Sarah J. Zaman, MBBS, PhD, FRACP, FCSANZ, SCAI-ELM[b],
Sonya N. Burgess, MBChB, PhD, FRACP, FCSANZ, SCAI-ELM[c],*

KEYWORDS

- Complete revascularization • Cardiovascular death • Multivessel disease • Prognosis
- ST elevation myocardial infarction

KEY POINTS

- High-quality randomized controlled trials, meta-analyses, and real-world data registries all show a significant prognostic benefit with timely complete revascularization in ST elevation myocardial infarction (STEMI).
- Recent meta-analyses consistently demonstrate a cardiovascular mortality benefit with timely complete revascularization.
- No benefit for physiologic testing when compared with angiography alone has been demonstrated in trials of complete revascularization in STEMI.
- Rates of incomplete revascularization remain high in contemporary observational all-comers cohorts.

INTRODUCTION

For decades, advances in ST elevation myocardial infarction (STEMI) care have been driven by timely reperfusion of the occluded culprit vessel. More recently, however, the focus has shifted to revascularization of nonculprit vessels in STEMI patients. This review focuses on evidence-based management of STEMI in the setting of multivessel disease (MVD), highlighting contemporary studies evaluating the impact of CR.

BACKGROUND

Cardiovascular disease is the leading cause of death worldwide.[1] One-third of patients with acute coronary syndrome (ACS) present with STEMI,[2,3] and half of these STEMI patients have MVD.[4] Management strategies employed to treat STEMI patients have, over the past 50 years, unrecognizably changed. Advances have resulted primarily from timely reperfusion of the occluded culprit vessel. In the past decade, however, the importance of CR for

---

Funding: The authors have nothing to disclose and have no commercial or financial conflicts of interest.
[a] Department of Cardiology, University of Sydney and Nepean Hospital, Derby Street, Kingswood, New South Wales 2747, Australia; [b] Department of Cardiology, University of Sydney, Monash University and Westmead Hospital, Corner of Darcy Road, Westmead 2145, Australia; [c] University of New South Wales, University of Sydney, and Department of Cardiology, Nepean Hospital, Derby Street, Sydney, New South Wales 2747, Australia
* Corresponding author.
E-mail address: Sonya.Burgess@health.nsw.gov.au
Twitter: @drsonyaburgess (S.S.)

STEMI patients has become increasingly apparent.

Five landmark complete revascularization (CR) randomized controlled trials (RCTs),[5–9] 3 meta-analyses,[10–12] and studies of all-comers consecutive STEMI cohorts[13–19] all support early CR for STEMI patients. This review discusses the management of STEMI in the setting of MVD, with a focus on contemporary data and completeness of revascularization. It begins by outlining first principles of contemporary STEMI management and reviews current guideline-based recommendations for patients presenting with MVD. It discusses each landmark trial in detail, along with recently published meta-analyses and all-comers cohort data and the implications of these for current clinical practice.

CONTEMPORARY ST ELEVATION MYOCARDIAL INFARCTION MANAGEMENT

Current evidence-based medicine for STEMI patients includes timely reperfusion, radial access, drug-eluting stent (DES) use, and optimal medical therapy. Guidelines recommend primary PCI as the preferred reperfusion strategy in patients with STEMI within 12 hours of symptoms onset, if it can be provided in a timely fashion.[20,21] Reperfusion with fibrinolysis followed by early transfer to a PCI-capable center is recommended for those with significant delays to primary PCI centers. Radial access is recommended based on data demonstrating a mortality benefit for STEMI patients treated using radial access,[22,23] along with a decrease in bleeding, vascular complications and need for blood transfusion. Second-generation DESs are recommended because trials have demonstrated reductions in cardiac death, myocardial infarction (MI), stent thrombosis, and target vessel revascularization (TVR) with late-generation DESs compared with bare metal stent in STEMI cohorts.[24] Dual antiplatelet therapy using aspirin plus P2Y12 receptor antagonist therapy with ticagrelor or prasugrel also is recommended when primary PCI is employed, based on data demonstrating a mortality benefit, and reduced recurrent MI, cardiovascular death, and major adverse cardiovascular event (MACE) with these agents.[25,26]

Current Guidelines Recommendations for Multivessel Disease in ST Elevation Myocardial Infarction

Current American Heart Association and European guidelines support CR in selected patients. The most recently published American

guidelines recommend, in patients who are hemodynamically stable with STEMI and MVD, nonculprit PCI can be considered either at the time of primary PCI or as a planned staged procedure and classify this as a class IIb recommendation.[21] The most recently published European guidelines state, "revascularization of non-infarct-related artery lesions should be considered in STEMI patients with MVD, before hospital discharge.[20] Because the optimal timing of revascularization (immediate vs staged) has not been adequately investigated, no recommendation in favor of immediate versus staged multivessel PCI can be formulated"[20] and the European guidelines classify this as a class IIa recommendation. Both guidelines were written before the Complete versus Culprit-only Revascularization to Treat Multi-vessel Disease After Early PCI for STEMI (COMPLETE) trial, and before major meta-analyses, including COMPLETE trial data, were published.

Defining Incomplete Revascularization Using the Residual SYNTAX Score

There is no universal definition for CR; definitions vary among currently published RCTs (Table 1).[5–9] The residual synergy between percutaneous intervention with Taxus and cardiac surgery (SYNTAX) score (rSS) now is used commonly to define the completeness of revascularization; it is independently associated with poor prognosis,[13,15–18,27,28] and all nonocclusive stenoses greater or equal to 50% stenosed in vessels greater than 1.5 mm are included. A score of 0 indicates no angiographically significant disease, 1 to 8 a low burden of incomplete revascularization, and greater than 8 a high burden of incomplete revascularization.

DATA SUPPORTING CULPRIT-ONLY REVASCULARIZATION

Prior to the publication of 5 landmark RCTs[5–9] evaluating the impact of incomplete revascularization in STEMI, the guideline-endorsed approach to STEMI revascularization was culprit-only PCI unless cardiogenic shock was present.[29,30] This recommendation was based primarily on observational data[31] because historical data provided conflicting evidence for the benefit of immediate CR in STEMI patients.[29–34]

The strongest data supporting culprit-only treatment were from a large network meta-analysis[31] of 18 studies (n = 40,280) published by Vlaar and colleagues.[31] A majority of included studies used retrospective observational methodology (14/18). Investigators found an odds

Table 1
Summary of outcomes for landmark complete revascularization ST elevation myocardial infarction trial outcomes

Randomized Controlled Trial	N	Timing	Primary Endpoint	Hazard Ratio for Primary Endpoint	Hazard Ratio for Cardiac Mortality	Hazard Ratio for Myocardial Infarction	Follow-up (y)
PRAMI	465	Sim	CD, nonfatal MI, RA	0.35 (0.21–0.58)	0.34 (0.11–1.08)	0.32 (0.13–0.75)	1.9
CvLPRIT	296	Sim or Inpt	D, recurrent MI, HF, IDR	0.45 (0.24–0.84)	0.27 (0.06–1.32)	0.48 (0.09–2.62)	1
DANAMI-3-PRIMULTI	627	Inpt	D, nonfatal MI, IDR	0.56 (0.38–0.83)	(0.19–1.70)	0.94 (0.47–1.90)	2.3
COMPARE-ACUTE	885	Sim or <72 hr	D, MI, R[a], CVA	0.35 (0.22–0.55)	1.0 (0.25–4.01)	0.50 (0.22–1.13)	1
COMPLETE	4041	Inpt or <45 d	CD, MI	0.74 (0.60–0.91)	0.93 (0.65–1.32)	0.68 (0.53–0.86)	3

Definitions of CR of noninfarct arteries varied for each trial as follows: COMPARE-ACUTE, arteries greater than 50% stenosis positive on FFR; COMPLETE, vessels greater than or equal to 2.5 mm with greater than or equal to 70% stenosis or 50% to 69% stenosis and a positive FFR; CvLPRIT, greater than 70% stenosis in a single view or greater than 50% in multiple views; DANAMI-3-PRIMULTI, arteries greater than 2 mm with greater than 50% stenosis and also FFR positive or greater than 90% stenosis with angiography alone; and PRAMI, arteries with greater than 50% stenosis.

Abbreviations: CD, cardiac death; D, death; HF, heart failure; IDR, ischemia-driven revascularization; Inpt, inpatient; MI, Myocardial infarction; R, revascularization; RA, refractory angina; Sim, simultaneous nonculprit treatment.

[a] Does not include clinically indicated revascularization performed within 45 days.

ratio (OR) for mortality of 0.7 (95% CI, 0.46–1.14) when comparing culprit-only PCI to multivessel PCI (simultaneous and staged). They also compared simultaneous multivessel PCI to staged PCI (at any time post–index PCI) and found an OR for mortality of 7.60 (95% CI, 2.80–24.90) in favor of staged PCI. At this time, however, there was a paucity of RCT data. Among the 18 studies included in this meta-analysis, only 2 studies directly compared simultaneous and staged multivessel PCI in an RCT setting (a total of 222 patients, 0.6% of all included patients), both were under-powered and 1 did not have a comparator culprit-only arm. As a result, Vlaar and colleagues' meta-analysis, although large, was likely to have been significantly affected by usual practice. During the period studied (2001–2010), only the most vulnerable patients were selected for simultaneous multivessel PCI and few other STEMI-specific RCT data addressing this issue were available. This data gap was recognized, and several randomized trials were planned to address this issue. Vlaar and colleagues concluded, based on their meta-analysis, that simultaneous multivessel primary PCI should not be encouraged, a finding that supported guideline recommendations at the time of publication.

LANDMARK RANDOMIZED CONTROLLED TRIALS OF COMPLETE REVASCULARIZATION

Contemporary data for the treatment of MVD in STEMI are provided by 5 landmark RCTs. These trials are the Preventive Angioplasty in Acute Myocardial Infarction (PRAMI) trial,[5] the Complete versus Lesion-Only Primary PCI trial (CvLPRIT) trial,[6] the Danish Trial in Acute Myocardial Infarction–Primary PCI in Patients With ST-elevation Myocardial Infarction and Multivessel Disease: Treatment of Culprit Lesion Only or Complete Revascularization (DANAMI-3–PRIMULTI) trial,[7] the Comparison Between FFR-guided Revascularization Versus Conventional Strategy in Acute STEMI Patients with MVD (COMPARE-ACUTE) trial,[8] and the COMPLETE trial.[9]

All compared complete revascularization to culprit-only revascularization in STEMI patients. All had differing primary composite endpoints but all report hazard ratios (HRs) of between 0.35 and 0.74 favoring CR. In 2 of the trials, significant differences also were seen for the combined endpoint of cardiac death and MI.[5,9] None of these trials have individually found a

cardiovascular mortality benefit for CR. Details of major findings from each trial are summarized in Table 1.

The PRAMI Trial
The PRAMI trial,[5] published in 2013, was the first of these 5 landmark RCTs studying CR in STEMI. This trial included 465 STEMI patients with MVD from 5 centers in the United Kingdom and compared outcomes in patients randomized to either multivessel PCI or to culprit vessel–only PCI. All nonculprit PCIs were performed during the index procedure. The trial was stopped early by the data safety and monitoring committee because a clear benefit was demonstrated with CR. The primary endpoint was a composite of death from cardiac causes, MI, or refractory angina, with a median follow-up of 23 months. The primary endpoint occurred in 9% (21/234) patients treated with multivessel PCI group and 22% (53/231) patients receiving culprit vessel PCI only (HR 0.35; 95% CI, 0.21–0.58; P < .001).[5] HRs for cardiac death, nonfatal MI, and cardiac death or nonfatal MI, respectively, were 0.34 (95% CI, 0.11–1.08), 0.32 (95% CI, 0.13–0.75), and 0.36 (95% CI, 0.18–0.73).

The CvLPRIT Trial
The CvLPRIT trial,[6] published in 2015, was the smallest of the 5 landmark RCTs, enrolling 296 STEMI patients and randomizing patients to either culprit-only PCI or multivessel PCI from 7 centers in the United Kingdom. Those randomized to multivessel PCI all were treated within the same hospital admission; a majority of patients (64%) had CR at the time of index PCI, the remainder (36%) had staged PCI in the same hospital admission. The primary endpoint was a composite all-cause death, MI, heart failure, or ischemia-driven revascularization within 12 months. The primary endpoint occurred in 10% (15/150) of patients in the CR group and 21% (31/146) randomized to culprit vessel–only PCI (HR 0.49; 95% CI, 0.24–0.84; P = .009).[6] HRs for cardiac death and MI, respectively, were 0.27 (95% CI, 0.06–1.32) and 0.48 (95% CI, 0.09–2.62). HRs for the composite of cardiac death and MI were not reported.

The DANAMI-3–PRIMULTI Trial
The DANAMI3-PRIMULTI[7] trial was the first of the 5 landmark RCTs to use fractional flow reserve (FFR)-guided revascularization of nonculprit lesion stenoses and was published in 2015. Enrolling 627 STEMI patients from 2 centers in Denmark, DANAMI-3–PRIMULTI patients were randomized to either culprit-only PCI or FFR-

guided CR performed 2 days after primary PCI and were followed for a mean of 2.3 years. The composite primary endpoint was all-cause mortality, MI, or ischemia-driven revascularization of nonculprit lesions. The primary endpoint occurred in 13% (40/314) of patients with (FFR-guided) CR and in 22% (68/313) of patients randomized to culprit lesion–only PCI (HR 0.56; 95% CI, 0.38–0.83; P = .004).[7] HRs for cardiac death, nonfatal MI, and cardiac death or nonfatal MI were, respectively, 0.56 (95% CI, 0.19–1.70), 0.94 (95% CI, 0.47–1.90), and 0.80 (95% CI, 0.45–1.45). The DANAMI-3–PRIMULTI trial outcomes favored CR but in this FFR-guided trial the magnitude of benefit for CR, when guided by FFR, was not as large as that in the similarly sized PRAMI trial, which used earlier PCI and angiographic assessment only.

The COMPARE-ACUTE Trial
The COMPARE-ACUTE trial,[8] published in 2017, randomized 885 STEMI patients with MVD to either culprit-only revascularization or FFR-guided CR using a 2:1 randomization strategy and was a multicenter trial enrolling patients from Europe and Asia. Of those patients randomized to CR, 83% had their nonculprit vessel treated at the time of the index procedure, with the remaining 27% of patients undergoing inpatient staged procedures, all performed within 72 hours (mean of 2.1 days for staged patients). All patients with lesions greater than or equal to 50% stenosis underwent FFR; however, FFR values were disclosed only in patients randomized to CR group. Clinically indicated elective revascularizations performed less than or equal to 45 days post–primary PCI were not counted as events in the culprit-only group. The primary endpoint was a composite of death, MI, revascularization, or cerebrovascular accident (CVA) at 12 months. The primary endpoint occurred in 7.8% (23/295) patients in the (FFR-guided) CR group and 20.5% (121/590) of patients randomized to culprit-only PCI (HR 0.35; 95% CI, 0.22–0.55; P < .001).[18] HRs for cardiac death and MI were, respectively, 1.00 (95% CI, 0.25–4.01) and 0.50 (95% CI, 0.22–1.13). HRs for the composite of cardiac death and MI were not reported. This FFR-guided trial had an almost identical magnitude of benefit to the PRAMI trial (when assessing HRs of their composite primary endpoints), both trials primarily employed simultaneous rather than staged PCI for nonculprit disease. The signal for improved rates of cardiac death or MI found, however, in the PRAMI trial was not evident among COMPARE-ACUTE trial patients.

The COMPLETE Trial
The COMPLETE trial,[9] published in 2019, was the largest of the 5 landmark CR RCTs. This multinational trial lead by North American investigators randomized 4041 STEMI patients with MVD to culprit vessel–only PCI or to CR either at the time of index hospitalization or following discharge. It was the only trial to use hard clinical endpoints of cardiac death and MI as a primary endpoint and the only trial to report rSSs. This trial also was the only trial to allow PCI of the nonculprit stenosis later than 5 days. The timing of CR was not randomized; a majority of patients received inpatient CR (68%); 84% had treatment within 3 weeks. FFR assessment was infrequent (<1%). There were 2 coprimary outcomes: the first was a composite of cardiac death or MI and the second a composite of cardiovascular death, MI, or ischemia-driven revascularization, with a mean follow-up of 3 years.

The composite endpoint of cardiac death or MI occurred in 7.8% (158/2016) of patients treated with CR and 10.5% (213/2025) of patients treated with culprit-only PCI (HR 0.74; 95% CI, 0.60–0.91); when ischemia-driven revascularization was included in this composite endpoint, rates were 8.9% (179/2016) and 16.7% (339/2025), respectively (HR 0.51; 95% CI, 0.43–0.61). HRs for cardiac death and MI alone were, respectively, 0.93 (95% CI, 0.65–1.32), and 0.68 (95% CI, 0.53–0.86). There was an expectation that the COMPLETE trial, due to its size, also would demonstrate a cardiovascular mortality benefit between randomized groups. Although differences in the primary endpoint were evident, no difference in cardiovascular death rates was observed, likely due in part to the low burden of disease among recruited patients, with median rSS scores of 7 in patients treated with culprit-only PCI.[9]

META-ANALYSES OF COMPLETE REVASCULARIZATION TRIALS

Since the publication of the COMPLETE trial, several meta-analyses have been published.[10–12] These meta-analyses consistently demonstrate a cardiac mortality benefit with timely CR.

The first of these meta-analyses was published by Pavasini and colleagues[11] and found an HR for cardiac death in STEMI patients receiving CR of 0.62 (95% CI, 0.39–0.97) and a number needed to treat to prevent 1 cardiovascular death of 70. In 2020, Bainey and colleagues[10] published a similar meta-analysis. This meta-analysis reported an OR for cardiovascular mortality with CR of 0.69 (95% CI, 0.48–

0.99). Data from a third meta-analysis from Chacko and colleagues[12] found similar results for STEMI patients randomized to CR reporting an HR for cardiovascular death of 0.68 (95% CI, 0.47–0.98).

ALL-COMERS ST ELEVATION MYOCARDIAL INFARCTION COHORTS

Data from RCTs and meta-analyses of RCTs, as described previously, provide the strongest evidence to date for CR. All-comers cohort data[9,13–19] further validate these findings and suggest the prognostic penalty for incomplete revascularization in unselected all-comers cohorts may be even greater than those demonstrated by RCT data.[9] Incomplete revascularization remains common in contemporary STEMI cohorts.[9,13–19,28] New York STEMI registry data found 78% of STEMI patients received incomplete revascularization[14]; Australian STEMI data found 75% of patients received incomplete revascularization (rSS $\geq$1).[13] A high burden of residual disease was seen in STEMI patients; rSSs of greater than 8 were present in 33% STEMI patients and in 58% of patients presenting with MVD.[13,19]

Incomplete revascularization in these studies (and similar studies[15,18]) are associated with higher rates of cardiac death and all-cause death; higher rates of hard composite clinical endpoints, such as cardiac death and MI; and higher rates of commonly used composite clinical endpoints, such as MACE. After multivariable risk adjustment, HRs for cardiac death and MI for STEMI patients with a high burden of residual disease (rSS >8) were 5.05 (2.27–11.26) compared with those with CR. After multivariate analysis HRs for cardiac death and MI for patients with incomplete revascularization with a low burden of disease (rSS 1–8) were 2.96 (95% CI, 1.31–6.69) compared with those with CR.[13] In unselected real-world STEMI cohorts with rSSs greater than 8 cardiac death or MI rates and cardiovascular death rates are 2-fold to 4-fold higher than those receiving culprit-only revascularization in recent RCTs.[9,13,15,18]

INCOMPLETE REVASCULARIZATION IN HIGH-RISK COHORTS
Complete Revascularization in ST Elevation Myocardial Infarction in the Setting of Cardiogenic Shock
Prior to 2017, guidelines for managing STEMI with MVD in the setting of cardiogenic shock were based primarily on observational registry data.[29,35] These data suggested that immediate CR improved in-hospital mortality and ischemic burden. RCT data, however, were lacking. The multicenter randomized Culprit Lesion Only PCI Versus Multivessel PCI in Cardiogenic Shock (CULPRIT-SHOCK) trial[36] addressed this data gap, comparing a culprit lesion–only strategy to immediate CR in STEMI patients present with cardiogenic shock. Thiele and colleagues[36] found a significant reduction in the primary endpoint of 30-day mortality or renal replacement therapy with culprit-only PCI versus immediate CR, 45.9% (158/344) compared with 55.4% (189/341) (relative risk [RR] 0.83; 95% CI, 0.71–0.96; $P = .01$) (driven by differences in 30-day mortality). As a result of the CULPRIT-SHOCK trial, in 2017 guidelines were revised; ESC[20,37] and American Heart Association[38] guidelines reversed previous recommendations and guidelines now do not recommend routine immediate multivessel PCI in shock (class IIIB). New post hoc analysis also has shown, however, that CR was achieved in 1 of 4 patients[28] and showed that rSS also is associated independently with poor prognosis in patients with cardiogenic shock,[28] suggesting further research is warranted.

Incomplete Revascularization in Women
There is a paucity of RCT data investigating the impact of incomplete revascularization in women, exacerbated by low representation of women in ACS trials. Outcomes post-STEMI are poorer for women than men and these outcome differences remain significant post–multivariable risk adjustment.[16,39–42] All-comers data suggest the prognostic penalty of incomplete revascularization may be even greater among high-risk cohorts, including women and diabetic patients.[16,17,19] Burgess and colleagues[16] found gender-based outcome differences are disproportionately observed among patients with a high burden of incomplete revascularization, whereas little gender-based outcome disparity is observed in patients with a low burden of disease (rSS $\leq$8). HRs for cardiac death or MI post-STEMI for women with a high burden of incomplete revascularization (rSS >8) were 2.14 (95% CI, 1.17–3.91) compared with men with men with the same rSSs and remained significant post–multivariable risk adjustment. Among women with incomplete revascularization (rSS >8), observed rates of cardiac death were 7.1%/year, in contrast to observed rates in men of 2.5%/year in men with rSS greater than 8 (HR 3.25; 95% CI, 1.41–7.51).[16] These data suggest improving overall rates of CR among STEMI patients also may help decrease gender-based outcome disparities.

Incomplete Revascularization in Patients with Diabetes

There are no RCT STEMI trials specifically studying outcomes for diabetic patients. Patients with diabetes also appear to be under-represented in earlier randomized trials.[17,19] All-comers observational data have demonstrated a higher risk for STEMI patients with diabetes than nondiabetic patients with STEMI.[17,19] Burgess and colleagues[17] reported HRs for cardiac death in STEMI patients with incomplete revascularization and diabetes of 2.66 (95% CI, 1.17–6.08) compared with nondiabetic patients with incomplete revascularization and report an adjusted HR for cardiac death of 1.94 (95% CI, 1.17–3.23) when comparing cardiac death rates in STEMI patients with MVD and diabetes to nondiabetic STEMI patients with MVD.[19] Burgess and colleagues[17] reported patients with incomplete revascularization and diabetes accounted for only 8% of STEMI patients but 30% of all cardiac deaths. These very high event rates suggest extrapolating results from lower-risk STEMI populations may result in an underestimation of risk for incompletely revascularized patients with diabetes and other high-risk cohorts.[17,19]

THE ROLE OF PHYSIOLOGIC ASSESSMENT WITH FRACTIONAL FLOW RESERVE

Among landmark trials of CR, 2 trials[7,8] mandated physiologic assessment using FFR assessment. These trials reported HR for their primary endpoints that were similar to those in landmark trials using angiographic assessment only (see Table 1). Bainey and colleagues[10] also assessed physiology testing versus angiographic assessment only among 10 CRs in STEMI trials and found no heterogeneity in cardiac death and MI rates when comparing trials using an angiography-guided strategy (OR 0.61; 95% CI, 0.38–0.97) versus FFR-guided strategy (OR 0.78; 95% CI, 0.43–1.44]; P int = 0.52). These data suggest no additional benefit of FFR during CR of STEMI patients.[10]

This finding is in contrast to results of the Fractional Flow Reserve Versus Angiography for Multivessel Evaluation Trial (FAME) trial[43] and the FAME II trial,[44] which have established a clear role for physiologic testing in more stable cohorts, because PCI based on angiographic severity alone can either underestimate or overestimate the severity of a coronary stenosis and, as a result, expose patients to unnecessary harm without significant benefit. FFR in STEMI patients, however, has been controversial. The role of microvascular obstruction in the culprit and watershed territories and abnormal vascular tone were hypothesized to increase the risk of both false-negative and false-positive measurements in the setting of STEMI.[7] Data from Ntalianis and colleagues,[45] however, do not support this theory. Ntalianis and colleagues[45] found FFR assessment of nonculprit arteries at the time of STEMI do not significantly differ from recovery FFR measurements and as such can be assessed in an acute setting.

It is likely that the lack of observed benefit for FFR in STEMI over angiographic assessment is due not to inaccuracies of measurement in the setting of STEMI but to the role of nonculprit vulnerable plaques, thin cap fibroadenoma, and the destabilizing proinflammatory milieu following STEMI,[46] where the degree of the stenosis may be less important than the stability of the lesion itself. In this setting imaging modalities, such as optimal coherence tomography (OCT), may prove a more useful tool. Contrast use and time associated with multivessel OCT, however, may limit applicability of OCT in the setting of STEMI. Lesion evaluation with FFR does not assess plaque stability. This may explain the absence of a significant incremental benefit in outcome with FFR versus angiographic assessment of nonculprit lesions. Data from the small OCT substudy of the COMPLETE trial[9] support this hypothesis.[47] This substudy included 93 patients from the COMPLETE trial and 425 lesions and found 47.3% of the patients had a nonculprit lesion with vulnerable plaque morphology.[47] Mehta and colleagues[9] hypothesized that this finding may explain the benefit of routine CR in patients with MVD and STEMI.

TIMING OF COMPLETE REVASCULARIZATION

The best timing for CR in STEMI is not yet clear. Currently, there are no adequately powered randomized data; trials evaluating the safety of delayed staging, NCT03135275 and NCT03621501, are awaited. In the COMPLETE trial, in 64% of cases, operators selected inpatient staging; in all other landmark RCTs, immediate or inpatient staging was mandated.[17] Thus, only 9% (596/6314) of all studied patients in these trials were treated with outpatient CR and only 2% (149/6314) of all patients enrolled in these landmark trials received PCI later than 34 days.[5–9]

The COMPLETE trial in particular must be read carefully; it clearly demonstrated the superiority of CR compared with culprit-only revascularization but it does not provide adequate data to support outpatient staged CR for all patients.[9] Cardiologists must be cognizant that although the COMPLETE trial allowed outpatient staging, the treating doctor selected the timing after assessing the patient and anatomy. Investigators of the trial carefully state, "We did not directly compare index hospitalization non-culprit lesion PCI and after-discharge nonculprit PCI as the timing was not randomly allocated." The COMPLETE trial article also states nonculprit PCI during primary PCI was not evaluated; as a result, a patient receiving 2-vessel PCI at the index procedure could be randomized to and classified as "culprit-only PCI" (that is, patients who received simultaneous nonculprit PCI at the time of the index procedure were eligible for enrollment and subsequently could be randomized to culprit-only PCI despite receiving some nonculprit PCI).

To date, the lowest HRs seen in landmark trials of compete revascularization are seen in the RCTs with the shortest time to CR, and the highest HRs are observed where the time to CR is prolonged (see Table 1).

The only meta-analysis to date to demonstrate an all-cause mortality benefit (rather than a cardiovascular mortality benefit) for CR found the all-cause mortality benefit was evident only in those with the earliest treatment. This meta-analysis by Pasceri and colleagues,[48] published in 2018, compared outcomes in RCT trial patients and compared early nonculprit PCI (defined as trials where >50% of patients were treated during the index procedure) to staged nonculprit PCI (>50% staged, from 2 days to 0 days; median 7.1 days). Early revascularization was associated with a significant reduction in risk for total mortality (RR 0.62; 95% CI, 0.39–0.97; $P = .03$) whereas staged revascularization did not demonstrate a significant all-cause mortality benefit (RR 1.02; 95% CI, 0.65–1.62; $P = .87$). Both showed a decrease in all-cause death or MI, but a larger benefit was seen with early CR: RR 0.53 (95% CI, 0.38–0.74) for early nonculprit PCI compared with RR 0.76 (95% CI, 0.58–0.99) for staged nonculprit PCI at 2 days to 20 days (median 7.1 days).

Currently, data from all landmark RCTs studying CR favor early CR; until further data prove otherwise, timely inpatient CR remains the safest evidence-based strategy. All-comers data also support this statement. Significant differences in rates of cardiac death and MI are seen between patients with incomplete revascularization and CR by less than or equal to 30 days, Kaplan-Meier event curves diverge early in these STEMI cohorts.[9,13–17]

RISKS OF COMPLETE REVASCULARIZATION

The potential risks of CR, in particular simultaneous or very early CR, also must be considered. As discussed previously for some cohorts, such as those with cardiogenic shock, the risks of immediate CR outweigh the benefits.

The potential risks of CR include increased exposure to contrast and the concurrent risk of renal failure or dialysis, increased radiation dose, and risks of a prolonged procedure and higher potential risk of complications. Concerns regarding these risks may in part explain variations in practice and a degree of treatment inertia regarding nonculprit disease observed in real-world cohorts.[13–17,19]

Four of the landmark trials overtly report several of these safety endpoints. In the CvLPRIT trial, there was no significant difference between groups in rates of contrast-induced nephropathy, major bleeding, or CVA.[49] In the DANAMI-3–PRIMULTI,[7] there was no significant difference between groups in the rates of contrast-induced nephropathy, stroke, or periprocedural MI. In the COMPARE-ACUTE trial,[8] there was no significant difference in major bleeding, any bleeding, or stent thrombosis. Contrast-induced nephropathy was not assessed, but investigators did report net adverse clinical event rates (cardiac death, MI, revascularization, CVA, and major bleeding) with an HR of 0.25 (95% CI, 0.16–0.38) favoring CR. In the COMPLETE trial,[9] no difference was found in rates of contrast-induced nephropathy, major bleeding, stent thrombosis, or stroke between groups. In combination, these data suggest even when both major risks and major benefits are considered among RCT-eligible patients, the risks of timely CR do not outweigh the benefits.

CONCLUSIONS AND FUTURE DIRECTIONS

There is now strong evidence demonstrating the importance of timely CR for STEMI patients. Data from numerous high-RCTs, contemporary meta-analyses, registry, and all-comers cohorts consistently show superior outcomes for patients offered timely CR. These studies no longer simply demonstrate a benefit for MACE but also now have demonstrated a benefit in hard clinical endpoints, including cardiovascular death and MI, with pooled data also showing a significant reduction in cardiovascular death. In combination, the strength and quality of these data support revision of guideline recommendations from the current class IIa or class IIb recommendations to class IA recommendations in future guidelines.

Data from CR RCTs and meta-analyses have addressed many therapeutic questions; however, several data gaps also remain. To date, no benefit for FFR assessment of nonculprit lesions in STEMI currently has been demonstrated; current data suggest plaque morphology rather than degree of stenosis may be of greater importance in STEMI cohorts. Further data regarding best timing of CR still are needed; current evidence for the benefit of CR is provided by studies where the great majority of patients received very early CR within days of the index event. As a result, until further data prove otherwise, timely inpatient CR remains the safest evidence-based strategy for most patients. For diabetic patients and for women, all-comers data suggest the prognostic penalty associated with incomplete revascularization may be even greater; however, adequately powered RCTs studying these patients also are needed.

The risks of immediate CR for patients with cardiogenic shock are high; these STEMI patients have clear RCT-based data demonstrating the importance of deferring nonculprit PCI to avoid harm. For all other cohorts, however, current RCT data demonstrate, even when both major risks and major benefits are considered, the benefits of timely CR significantly outweigh the risks.

LIMITATIONS

Current data have yet to demonstrate an all-cause mortality benefit for CR for all patients. An all-cause mortality benefit has been demonstrated only in CR trials with simultaneous or very early CR. Careful evaluation of individual patient risk also is warranted. For patients who would not meet the inclusion criteria of the landmark RCT trials discussed in this review, a balanced approach addressing both potential risks and likely benefits of CR is suggested.

SUMMARY

Current data indicate the superiority of timely CR over culprit-only revascularization in patients with MVD without cardiogenic shock. These data, drawn from high-quality RCTs and meta-analyses, also are supported by real-world data registries. A cardiovascular mortality benefit for timely CR in STEMI now has been demonstrated by several meta-analyses. The prognostic penalty of incomplete revascularization in STEMI is clear, but rates of incomplete revascularization remain high in contemporary observational all-comers cohorts. Strategies designed to decrease rates of incomplete revascularization for STEMI patients are needed. Further guideline revision accounting for more recent RCTs and meta-analyses and quality improvement initiatives may be required.

CLINICS CARE POINTS

- Complete revascularization should be a priority when managing STEMI patients.
- Incomplete revascularization is common in STEMI patients with multivessel disease.
- Complete revascularization is prognostically important and associated with significantly lower rates of cardiac death.
- A residual syntax score > 8 is associated with very high rates of cardiac death and major adverse cardiac events.
- For women and for diabetic patients with incomplete revascularization the prognostic penalty associated with incomplete revascularization is even greater.
- Current evidence for the benefit of complete revascularization is provided by studies where the great majority of patients receive very early CR within days of the index event.
- Timely inpatient CR remains the safest evidence-based strategy for most patients until further RCT studies randomizing the timing of non-culprit CR are published.

REFERENCES

1. World Health Organization. Global Health Estimates 2016: Deaths by Cause, Age, Sex, by Country and by Region, 2000-2016. Geneva, World Health Organization; 2018.
2. O'Gara PT, Kushner FG, Ascheim DD, et al. 2013 ACCF/AHA guideline for the management of ST-elevation myocardial infarction: a report of the American College of Cardiology Foundation/American Heart Association Task Force on Practice Guidelines. J Am Coll Cardiol 2013;61:e78–140.
3. Muller DW, Topol EJ, Ellis SG, et al. Multivessel coronary artery disease: a key predictor of short-term prognosis after reperfusion therapy for acute myocardial infarction. Thrombolysis and Angioplasty in Myocardial Infarction (TAMI) Study Group. Am Heart J 1991;121:1042–9.

4. Park DW, Clare RM, Schulte PJ, et al. Extent, location, and clinical significance of non-infarct-related coronary artery disease among patients with ST-elevation myocardial infarction. JAMA 2014;312:2019–27.

5. Wald DS, Morris JK, Wald NJ, et al. Randomized trial of preventive angioplasty in myocardial infarction. N Engl J Med 2013;369:1115–23.

6. Gershlick AH, Khan JN, Kelly DJ, et al. Randomized trial of complete versus lesion-only revascularization in patients undergoing primary percutaneous coronary intervention for stemi and multivessel disease: The CvLPRIT trial. J Am Coll Cardiol 2015;65:963–72.

7. Engstrøm T, Kelbæk H, Helqvist S, et al, DANAMI-3—PRIMULTI Investigators. Complete revascularisation versus treatment of the culprit lesion only in patients with ST-segment elevation myocardial infarction and multivessel disease (DANAMI-3 — PRIMULTI): an open-label , randomised controlled trial. Lancet 2015;386:665–71.

8. Smits PC, Abdel-Wahab M, Neumann F-J, et al. Fractional flow reserve–guided multivessel angioplasty in myocardial infarction. N Engl J Med 2017;376:1234–44.

9. Mehta SR, Wood DA, Storey RF, et al. Complete revascularization with multivessel PCI for myocardial infarction. N Engl J Med 2019;381:1411–21.

10. Bainey KR, Engstrøm T, Smits PC, et al. Complete vs culprit-lesion-only revascularization for ST-segment elevation myocardial infarction. JAMA Cardiol 2020;75:1–9.

11. Pavasini R, Biscaglia S, Barbato E, et al. Complete revascularization reduces cardiovascular death in patients with ST-segment elevation myocardial infarction and multivessel disease: systematic review and meta-analysis of randomized clinical trials. Eur Heart J 2019;41(42):4103–10.

12. Chacko L, Howard JP, Rajkumar C, et al. Effects of percutaneous coronary intervention on death and myocardial infarction stratified by stable and unstable coronary artery disease: a meta-analysis of randomized controlled trials. Circ Cardiovasc Qual Outcomes 2020;13:1–15.

13. Burgess SN, French JK, Nguyen TL, et al. The impact of incomplete revascularization on early and late outcomes in ST-elevation myocardial infarction. Am Heart J 2018;205:31–41.

14. Hannan EL, Zhong Y, Berger PB, et al. Association of coronary vessel characteristics with outcome in patients with percutaneous coronary interventions with incomplete revascularization. JAMA Cardiol 2018;3:123–30.

15. Galvão C, Cid-alvarez AB, Redondo A, et al. Prognostic impact of residual SYNTAX score in patients with ST-elevation myocardial infarction and multivessel disease: analysis of an 8-year all-comers registry. Int J Cardiol 2017;243:21–6.

16. Burgess SN, Juergens CP, Nguyen TL, et al. Comparison of late cardiac death and myocardial infarction rates in women vs men with st-elevation myocardial infarction. Am J Cardiol 2020;128:120–6.

17. Burgess SN, Juergens CP, Nguyen T, et al. Diabetes and incomplete revascularisation in ST elevation myocardial infarction. Hear Lung Circ 2020.

18. Loutfi M, Ayad S, Sobhy M. Impact of the residual SYNTAX score on outcomes of revascularization in patients with st-segment elevation myocardial infarction and multivessel disease. Clin Med Insights Cardiol.2016;10:29–35.

19. Burgess S, Juergens CP, Yang W, et al. Cardiac mortality, diabetes mellitus, and multivessel disease in ST elevation myocardial infarction. Int J Cardiol 2021;323:13–8.

20. Ibanez B, James S, Agewall S, et al. 2017 ESC Guidelines for the management of acute myocardial infarction in patients presenting with ST-segment elevation. Eur Heart J 2018;39:119–77.

21. Levine GN, Bates ER, Blankenship JC, et al. 2015 ACC/AHA/SCAI Focused Update on Primary Percutaneous Coronary Intervention for Patients with ST-Elevation Myocardial Infarction An Update of the 2011 ACCF/AHA/SCAI Guideline for Percutaneous Coronary Intervention and the 2013 ACCF/AHA Guideline for th. J Am Coll Cardiol 2016;67:1235–50.

22. Romagnoli E, Biondi-Zoccai G, Sciahbasi A, et al. Radial versus femoral randomized investigation in ST-segment elevation acute coronary syndrome: the RIFLE-STEACS (Radial Versus Femoral Randomized Investigation in ST-Elevation Acute Coronary Syndrome) study. J Am Coll Cardiol 2012;60:2481–9.

23. Valgimigli M, Frigoli E, Leonardi S, et al. Radial versus femoral access and bivalirudin versus unfractionated heparin in invasively managed patients with acute coronary syndrome (MATRIX): final 1-year results of a multicentre, randomised controlled trial. Lancet 2018;392:835–48.

24. Palmerini T, Biondi-Zoccai G, Della Riva D, et al. Clinical outcomes with drug-eluting and bare-metal stents in patients with ST-segment elevation myocardial infarction. J Am Coll Cardiol 2013;62:496–504.

25. Wallentin L, Becker RC, Budaj A, et al. Ticagrelor versus clopidogrel in patients with acute coronary syndromes. N Engl J Med 2009;361:1045–57.

26. Wiviott SD, Braunwald E, McCabe CH, et al. Prasugrel versus clopidogrel in patients with acute coronary syndromes. N Engl J Med 2007;357:2001–15.

27. Généreux P, Palmerini T, Caixeta A, et al. Quantification and impact of untreated coronary artery disease after percutaneous coronary intervention: the residual SYNTAX (Synergy Between PCI with Taxus

and Cardiac Surgery) score. J Am Coll Cardiol 2012;59:2165–74.

28. Barthélémy O, Rouanet S, Brugier D, et al. Predictive value of the residual SYNTAX score in patients with cardiogenic shock. J Am Coll Cardiol 2021;77: 144–55.

29. Levine GN, Bates ER, Blankenship JC, et al. 2011 ACCF/AHA/SCAI Guideline for Percutaneous Coronary Intervention: a report of the American College of Cardiology Foundation/American Heart Association Task Force on Practice Guidelines and the Society for Cardiovascular Angiography and Interventions. Circulation 2011;124: e574–651.

30. Hamm CW, Bassand J-P, Agewall S, et al. ESC Guidelines for the management of acute coronary syndromes in patients presenting without persistent ST-segment elevation: The Task Force for the management of acute coronary syndromes (ACS) in patients presenting without persistent ST-segment elevatio. Eur Heart J 2011;32:2999–3054.

31. Vlaar PJ, Mahmoud KD, Holmes DR, et al. Culprit vessel only versus multivessel and staged percutaneous coronary intervention for multivessel disease in patients presenting with ST-segment elevation myocardial infarction. J Am Coll Cardiol 2011;58: 692–703.

32. Bhindi R, Banning AP. Not So Fast. Circulation 2017;135:1574–6.

33. Mauri L. Nonculprit lesions innocent-or guilty by association. N Engl J Med 2013;369:1166–7.

34. Corpus RA, House JA, Marso SP, et al. Multivessel percutaneous coronary intervention in patients with multivessel disease and acute myocardial infarction. Am Heart J 2004;148:493–500.

35. Hussain F, Philipp RK, Ducas RA, et al. The ability to achieve complete revascularization is associated with improved in-hospital survival in cardiogenic shock due to myocardial infarction: Manitoba cardiogenic shock registry investigators. Catheter Cardiovasc Interv 2011;78:540–8.

36. Thiele H, Akin I, Sandri M, et al. One-year outcomes after PCI strategies in cardiogenic shock. N Engl J Med 2018;379:1699–710.

37. Ibanez B, Halvorsen S, Roffi M, et al. Integrating the results of the CULPRIT-SHOCK trial in the 2017 ESC ST-elevation myocardial infarction guidelines: viewpoint of the task force. Eur Heart J 2018;39:4239–42.

38. Thiele H, Desch S. CULPRIT-SHOCK (Culprit Lesion Only PCI Versus Multivessel Percutaneous Coronary Intervention in Cardiogenic Shock). Circulation 2018;137:1314–6.

39. Khan E, Brieger D, Amerena J, et al. Differences in management and outcomes for men and women with ST-elevation myocardial infarction. Med J Aust 2018;209:118–23.

40. Stehli J, Martin C, Brennan A, et al. Sex differences persist in time to presentation, revascularization, and mortality in myocardial infarction treated with percutaneous coronary intervention. J Am Heart Assoc 2019;8:1–9.

41. Heer T, Hochadel M, Schmidt K, et al. Sex differences in percutaneous coronary intervention—insights from the coronary angiography and PCI registry of the German Society of Cardiology. J Am Heart Assoc 2017;6:1–10.

42. Greenwood BN, Carnahan S, Huang L. Patient–physician gender concordance and increased mortality among female heart attack patients. Proc Natl Acad Sci U S A 2018;115(34):8569–74.

43. Tonino PAL, De Bruyne B, Pijls NHJ, et al. Fractional flow reserve versus angiography for guiding percutaneous coronary intervention. N Engl J Med 2009;360:213–24.

44. Fearon WF, Nishi T, De Bruyne B, et al. Clinical outcomes and cost-effectiveness of fractional flow reserve–guided percutaneous coronary intervention in patients with stable coronary artery disease. Circulation 2018;137:480–7.

45. Ntalianis A, Sels J-W, Davidavicius G, et al. Fractional flow reserve for the assessment of nonculprit coronary artery stenoses in patients with acute myocardial infarction. JACC Cardiovasc Interv 2010;3:1274–81.

46. Hansson GK, Libby P, Tabas I. Inflammation and plaque vulnerability. J Intern Med 2015;278:483–93.

47. Pinilla-Echeverri N, Mehta SR, Wang J, et al. Nonculprit Lesion Plaque Morphology in Patients With ST-Segment-Elevation Myocardial Infarction: Results From the COMPLETE Trial Optical Coherence Tomography Substudys. Circ Cardiovasc Interv 2020;13(7):e008768.

48. Pasceri V, Patti G, Pelliccia F, et al. Complete revascularization during primary percutaneous coronary intervention reduces death and myocardial infarction in patients with multivessel disease: meta-analysis and meta-regression of randomized trials. JACC Cardiovasc Interv 2018;11:833–43.

49. Kelly DJ, McCann GP, Blackman D, et al. Complete Versus culprit-Lesion only PRimary PCI Trial (CVLPRIT): a multicentre trial testing management strategies when multivessel disease is detected at the time of primary PCI: rationale and design. EuroIntervention 2013;8:1190–8.

Management of Cardiogenic Shock in Patients with Acute Myocardial Infarction

Katherine J. Kunkel, MD, MSEd[a], Brittany Fuller, MD[a],
Mir B. Basir, DO[b],*

KEYWORDS

- STEMI • Cardiogenic shock • Mechanical circulatory support
- Percutaneous coronary intervention

KEY POINTS

- Acute myocardial infarction and cardiogenic shock (AMI-CS) is associated with significant morbidity and mortality. The most common cause of AMI-CS is pump failure owing to left ventricular (LV) dysfunction.
- AMI-CS consists of multiple pathophysiologic subtypes; however, the final common pathway occurs with an ischemic insult resulting in reduced LV compliance leading to increased LV end-diastolic pressure, LV dilation, and reduced LV function. Compensatory tachycardia and peripheral vasoconstriction result in worsening myocardial ischemia, whereas the reduced LV function leads to worsening systemic hypotension and activation of inflammatory mediators. These physiologic derangements can culminate in multisystem organ failure and death.
- Early mechanical revascularization improves survival in such patents. Development of STEMI systems of care has increased the utilization of revascularization in AMI-CS from 19% in 2001 to 60% in 2014.
- Mechanical circulatory support devices are increasingly used to support and prevent hemodynamic collapse. Intra-aortic balloon pump counterpulsation has been found to have limited utility in AMI-CS, whereas more robust support devices, including VA-ECMO and Impella, are currently enrolling in large-scale randomized controlled trials to elicit their use in AMI-CS.
- Although these large-scales studies are being conducted, the use of shock protocols and teams has been associated with improved outcomes in AMI-CS.

BACKGROUND

Incidence and Historical Impact of Revascularization Strategies on Outcomes

Cardiogenic shock (CS) occurs in 5% to 10% of patients presenting with acute myocardial infarction (AMI).[1] Patients presenting with ST-elevation myocardial infarction (STEMI) are 2-fold more likely to present with CS than those presenting with non-STEMI (5.9% vs 2.9%).[2] CS is more common among patients ≥75 years old and women. In a large US registry examining patients presenting with STEMI and CS, 42.3% had an anterior STEMI, 38.6% had an inferior STEMI, and 19.1% had another culprit.[3]

Before early mechanical revascularization, the mortality rate for acute myocardial infarction and

---

[a] Henry Ford Health Care System, 2799 West Grand Boulevard (K-2 Cath Lab), Detroit, MI 48202, USA; [b] STEMI, Acute Mechanical Circulatory Support, Interventional Cardiology, Henry Ford Hospital, Henry Ford Health Care System, 2799 West Grand Boulevard (K-2 Cath Lab), Detroit, MI 48202, USA
* Corresponding author.
E-mail address: Mbasir1@hfhs.org

Intervent Cardiol Clin 10 (2021) 345–357
https://doi.org/10.1016/j.iccl.2021.03.006
2211-7458/21/© 2021 Elsevier Inc. All rights reserved.

cardiogenic shock (AMI-CS) was between 70% and 80%.[4] The "SHould we emergently revascularize Occluded Coronaries for cardiogenic shock" (SHOCK) trial demonstrated a reduction in mortality from 63.1% in medically managed patients to 50.3% in patients managed with early mechanical revascularization at 6 months.[5] This 13% absolute risk reduction in mortality persisted at 1 year.[6] Subsequent international registry data demonstrated marked improvements in mortality among patients with AMI-CS, with US-based registries demonstrating case fatality rates decreasing from 68% in 2001 to 38% in 2014. Through the development of STEMI networks, the use of PCI for STEMI in patients with CS increased from 19% to 60% between 2001 and 2014.

Independent predictors of mortality in AMI with CS include advanced age, Killip class IV on admission, low systolic blood pressure on admission, the diagnosis of STEMI, peripheral arterial disease, and stroke.[2] Multiple risk scores have been created using these and other clinical characteristics to identify patients at the highest risk for short- and long-term adverse outcomes.[7,8]

Definition of Cardiogenic Shock and Society for Coronary Angiography and Interventions Shock Stages

CS is a low-output state frequently leading to significant end-organ hypoperfusion. CS has been classically defined as a systolic blood pressure ≤90 mm Hg for ≥30 minutes or the need for vasopressors or mechanical circulatory support (MCS) devices to maintain a systolic blood pressure ≥90 mm Hg.[6,9] Definitions of CS also typically include the presence of end-organ hypoperfusion, variably defined as the presence of decreasing urine output, altered mental status, or an elevated serum lactate (>2.0 mmol/L), as well as hemodynamic parameters, such as the presence of a cardiac index ≤2.2 L/min/m², cardiac power output less than 0.6 W, and pulmonary capillary wedge pressure ≥15 mm Hg.[10] Although this definition does not address the spectrum of shock severity and does not take into account the cause of shock, it does serve as a starting point for identifying these high-risk patients.

Although the general diagnostic criteria for CS have been well established in the setting of clinical trials, before 2019, there was no uniform method for describing the various stages of CS severity. Variability in defining the severity of CS has limited comparison of outcomes across clinical trials.

In 2019, the consensus statement on the classification of CS was put forth by the Society for Coronary Angiography and Intervention (SCAI).[11] This schema uses a combination of biochemical markers, clinical findings, and hemodynamics to classify CS into one of 5 categories: A, "At Risk"; B, "Beginning"; C, "Classic"; D, "Deteriorating"; or E, "Extremis." Retrospective validation of the SCAI classification of CS has shown this categorization to be a robust predictor of in-hospital mortality among patients with CS (**Fig. 1**).[12]

Mechanism and Pathophysiology

The most common cause of CS in AMI is pump failure owing to left ventricular (LV) dysfunction. There are several mechanisms of AMI that can result in LV failure, systemic hypoperfusion, and shock.

- Patients can present with a large myocardial infarction (MI), resulting in significant stunning, ischemia, and infarction to a large area of myocardium, resulting in acute pump dysfunction, hypotension, and hemodynamic compromise.
- In patients with preexisting multivessel coronary artery disease, an AMI in a small or moderate territory may result in a large ischemic insult because of underlying disease in a noninfarct artery. For example, a patient with a chronically occluded left anterior descending (LAD) artery and an inferior MI can present with hemodynamic collapse, as the right coronary artery (RCA) frequently supplies collaterals to the LAD territory. Patients with multivessel disease similarly may develop global ischemia because of poor coronary perfusion in the setting of systemic hypotension and preexisting stenoses in non-infarct-related arteries.
- Patients with underlying cardiomyopathy can present with an ischemic insult, which may result in hemodynamic compromise because of baseline cardiac dysfunction with poor myocardial reserve and tenuous hemodynamics.
- Last, patients with AMI and prolonged cardiac arrest can develop rapid global end-organ hypoperfusion, often resulting in advanced stages of metabolic shock.

In all these pathophysiologic subtypes, the final common pathway occurs via the ischemic cascade in which reduced compliance of the LV is associated with increased LV end-diastolic

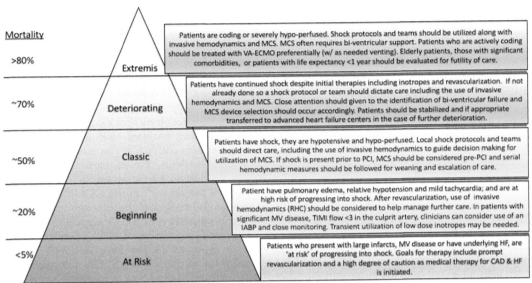

Fig. 1. SCAI classification of shock. CAD, coronary artery disease; HF, heart failure; MV, multi-vessel; RHC, right heart catheterization; TIMI, thrombolysis in myocardial infarction.

pressure, LV dilation, and reduced systolic function. Compensatory tachycardia and peripheral vasoconstriction further potentiate myocardial ischemia by increasing myocardial oxygen demand. Reduction in systolic function leads to further systemic hypotension, initiating a cascade of neurohormonal mediators that potentiates the hemodynamic and metabolic effects of CS. The release of catecholamines, vasopressin, and angiotensin II leads to peripheral vasoconstriction and sodium retention. Although this transiently improves coronary and peripheral perfusion, increased afterload and volume result in pulmonary edema and further exacerbation of cardiac dysfunction. In the 24 to 72 hours after MI, cytokine levels, including tumor necrosis factor-α, interleukin-6 procalcitonin, C-reactive protein, and others, have been shown to be elevated in patients with CS.[13] Patients in the late stages of CS develop a systemic inflammatory response characterized by low systemic vascular resistance progressing to vasodilatory shock. This physiology, seen in one-fifth of patients with AMI-CS, portends a 2-fold risk of death when adjusted for age.[14]

Right Ventricular Shock

Right ventricular (RV) infarction results in decreased RV compliance and contractile function. With acute dysfunction of the RV, the RV inadequately fills the LV, causing an acute reduction in cardiac output. As the failing RV dilates,

the interventricular dependence between the 2 ventricles is altered. Given the constraints of the pericardium, this adversely affects the performance of the LV, reducing cardiac output and decreasing LV compliance.[15]

RV infarctions are often accompanied by sinus bradycardia and atrioventricular block, particularly in proximal RCA occlusions, which involve the conus and atrioventricular nodal arteries. Up to one-third of patients with RV infarction also develop atrial fibrillation.[16]

Isolated RV infarction leading to CS is relatively rare, comprising 3% to 5% of cases.[17] Although RV infarction most commonly accompanies a posterior/inferior AMI, autopsy series have found that many proximal RCA infarctions do not result in significant RV necrosis.[18] The lack of RV necrosis has been attributed to reduced myocardial oxygen demand of the RV, given its lower muscle mass and an extensive collateral network from the left coronary system.

RV hypertrophy is postulated to be a predisposing factor to the development of RV infarction.[19] RV infarction is more common in patients who are younger, have single-vessel coronary artery disease, and are presenting with their first MI.[17]

There are conflicting data comparing the mortality among patients with predominant RV and LV shock. In the SHOCK trial registry, similar in-hospital mortality was reported among patients with CS because of isolated RV and LV infarction (53.1% for RV shock vs 60.8% for LV shock; $P = .296$).[17] In this study, there were relatively low rates of primary PCI among patients with CS, although among the 36% undergoing primary PCI, there was no difference in mortality among those with RV and LV shock (41.7% vs 46.2%). Contradictory data were presented by Brodie and colleagues that showed that in a single-center 20-year experience among 2496 consecutive patients with STEMI, the in-hospital mortality of shock owing to RV infarction was significantly lower than with LV infarction (23% vs 50%; $P = .01$). Shock because of RV infarction was an independent predictor of late cardiac survival.[20] Differences in these findings have been attributed to differences in methodologies, with the SHOCK registry selecting patients with more comorbidities and worse outcomes, consistent with an overall sicker cohort of patients.

RV infarction clinically manifests with the triad of hypotension, elevated jugular venous pressure, and clear lung fields. Several echocardiographic and hemodynamic parameters have been studied to characterize RV dysfunction in the setting of CS. In 2012, Korabathina and colleagues published a retrospective analysis of patients with inferior STEMI and suspected RV dysfunction compared with controls with acute coronary syndrome with left coronary stenting and with nonobstructive coronary disease. Three hemodynamic parameters (RA:PCWP ratio, calculated RV stroke work, and pulmonary artery [PA] pulsatility index [PAPi], where PAPi = PA pulse pressure/RA pressure) were found to correlate to echocardiographic findings of RV dysfunction as well as clinical outcomes. Of the parameters studied, PAPi was identified as having the highest sensitivity (88.9%) and specificity (98.3%) for identifying patients with severe RV dysfunction as defined by the combined endpoint of in-hospital mortality or need for percutaneous RV MCS.[21]

Biventricular Shock

RV infarction has been variably reported in association with LV infarction, with rates ranging from 14% to 84% in the literature.[17] In inferior/posterior infarctions, concomitant RV infarction has been described in up to 50% of cases. In addition, RV infarction has been described in up to 13% of anterior AMI.[18] Although biventricular heart failure can be identified noninvasively with the use of echocardiography and clinical presentation, right heart catheterization remains the gold standard for identifying biventricular failure. Use of hemodynamic parameters, including cardiac power output to identify the highest-risk patients for in-hospital mortality as well as PAPi and RA:PCWP ratio to quantify contribution of right heart dysfunction, can identify high-risk patients who may require biventricular MCS.[22]

Iatrogenic Cardiogenic Shock

Approximately 70% of patients with CS complicating AMI develops shock during their hospitalization. These patients have a higher mortality than patients with CS at the time of admission.[6] In some patients, the development of shock is due to hemodynamic stress of reperfusion or medical therapies.[23] In the COMMIT trial, intravenous (IV) metoprolol at the time of presentation in patients with STEMI was associated with increased incidence of CS.[24] Similar findings were reported in the SWEDEHEART registry, which found that among STEMI patients without CS, those given IV beta-blockers were more likely to develop CS and had higher in-hospital mortality.[25] In contemporary practice, early initiation of beta-blockers, opioids, ACE inhibitors, or diuretics in patients with marginal hemodynamics who are unable to tolerate changes in preload, afterload, inotropy, or chronotropy has been postulated to cause CS.

MANAGEMENT OF CARDIOGENIC SHOCK
Anticoagulation and Antiplatelet Agents

Patients presenting with STEMI and CS should routinely be given aspirin and heparin at the time of presentation. Controversy exists regarding the timing of P2Y12 inhibitor initiation and the agent of choice in patients with CS given concerns with reduced drug absorption and impaired hepatic metabolism of oral agents. Retrospective observational data have shown reduced efficacy of clopidogrel in CS.[26] Although no definitive conclusions can be drawn from the available data, IV antiplatelet agents, including cangrelor or glycoprotein IIb/IIIa inhibitors, may provide more reliable antiplatelet activity in the setting of CS. Use of IV agents must be weighed against increased risk of bleeding with these more potent antiplatelet agents, particularly among patients who may require large-bore arterial access for MCS.

Inotropes and Vasopressors

The dose of vasopressors and inotropes required to establish hemodynamic stability has been demonstrated to predict mortality in intensive care unit patients.[27] Increased myocardial oxygen consumption associated with inotropes and vasopressors use may negatively affect overall mortality in patients with AMI and CS.[28]

Understanding a patient's hemodynamic status and the mechanism of action of vasopressors and inotropes allows for tailored selection of vasoactive medications to optimize a patient's hemodynamic performance and restore tissue perfusion. The most commonly used vasoactive medications include dopamine, dobutamine, epinephrine, milrinone, norepinephrine, phenylephrine, and vasopressin (Table 1).

The hemodynamics associated with normotensive CS are a low stroke volume and cardiac output with an elevated systemic vascular resistance. In these cases, inodilators, such as dobutamine and milrinone, are the agents of choice. Multiple studies have demonstrated an association between inotrope use and in-hospital mortality, emphasizing the importance of using these agents as sparingly as possible.[29,30] Dobutamine generally results in greater inotropy with more arrhythmias and myocardial ischemia, whereas milrinone is associated with more significant vasodilation and hypotension.[31] Individualized selection based on the patient's hemodynamics and revascularization status is recommended in selecting inodilators in the setting of AMI-CS.

In states of CS with hypotension, inoconstrictors (eg, norepinephrine, epinephrine, and dopamine) are used to augment cardiac output and systemic vascular resistance. These endogenous catecholamines have variable levels of alpha-1 and beta-1 receptor stimulation, resulting in vasoconstriction and increased inotropy.

In general, norepinephrine is regarded as the first-line inoconstrictor over dopamine or epinephrine. A prospective randomized trial comparing norepinephrine to dopamine as a first-line pressor among patients with undifferentiated shock demonstrated similar mortality but higher rates of arrhythmias with dopamine versus norepinephrine.[32] In the subgroup with CS, dopamine was found to have statistically significantly higher rates of death and increased ischemic events. This was associated with increased ischemic events in the dopamine group. Subsequent observational data showed increased utilization of norepinephrine and decreased utilization of dopamine in the period between 2007 and 2015 among greater than 10,000 patients in a tertiary care center cardiac intensive care unit. After controlling for overall vasopressor and inotrope use and illness severity using a multivariable logistic regression model, norepinephrine was associated with lower in-hospital mortality compared with other vasopressors.[33]

Similarly, observational data have shown higher rates of mortality in patients with CS treated with epinephrine compared with other vasopressors in multivariate logistic regression analysis.[34] These results were confirmed in a meta-analysis of vasopressor use and outcomes in patients with CS. Patients treated with epinephrine had a higher incidence of short-term mortality, and after propensity matching, a 3-fold increase in the risk of death compared with patients treated with other vasopressors.[35]

The final vasoactive agents used in the management of CS are the vasoconstrictors phenylephrine and vasopressin. These medications have limited use in the management of CS and are generally reserved for low afterload states or when inotropy is harmful, such as with tachyarrhythmias or LV outflow tract obstruction.

Revascularization

The methods of revascularization in patients suffering from AMI-CS have undergone a steady evolution from early medical therapy with anticoagulation and thrombolysis to mechanical therapy with surgery or percutaneous coronary intervention (PCI). The goal of revascularization is to reduce infarct size, preserve LV function, and improve survival.

Early thrombolytic trials were successful in achieving infarct artery patency in approximately 50% to 70% of patients within 90 minutes of presentation. Thrombolysis, however, was inferior to primary percutaneous balloon angioplasty, which restored TIMI (thrombolysis in myocardial infarction) grade 3 coronary blood flow in 80% to 95% of patients.[36,37] Thrombolytic therapy has also been associated with complications, including bleeding requiring transfusion in 5% of patients and stroke in 1.8% of patients.[36] Despite thrombolytic therapy being relatively safe and effective, it has a limited effect on outcomes in patients presenting with AMI-CS, with a short-term mortality of greater than 70% in this group. Older age is the strongest predictor of worse outcomes among patients with AMI-CS treated with thrombolysis.[38,39] Despite these limitations, thrombolysis remains a viable option for reperfusion in patients in which timely mechanical intervention is not feasible.

By the early 2000s, several nonrandomized studies reported reduced mortality in patients with AMI-CS treated with primary PCI. These observational studies prompted the SHOCK trial, a well-known multicenter randomized controlled trial.[6] This trial compared emergency revascularization with initial medical stabilization in patients presenting with shock owing to LV failure complicating AMI. The survival benefit favoring mechanical revascularization was largest

Table 1
Inotropes and vasopressors

Drug	Typical Dosing	Receptor	CO	Effect SVR	PVR
Inodilator					
Milrinone	0.125–0.750 µg/kg/min	cAMP	↑↑↑	↓↓	↓↓
Dobutamine	2.5–10 µg/kg/min	α β1 β2	↑↑↑	↓	↓
Inoconstrictor					
Dopamine	1–4 µg/kg/min	D	↑	↓	
	5–10 µg/kg/min	α β1 D	↑↑	↔	
	10–20 µg/kg/min	α β1 D	↑	↑↑	↑
Epinephrine	1–20 µg/min	α β1 β2	↑↑	↑	
Norepinephrine	1–40 µg/min	α β1	↑	↑↑	
Vasoconstrictor					
Phenylephrine	40–180 µg/min	α	↔	↑↑↑	↑↑
Vasopressin	0.01–0.06 U/min	v1, v2	↔	↑↑↑	↓

Abbreviations: CO, cardiac output; PVR, pulmonary vascular resistance; SVR, systemic vascular resistance.

when revascularization was performed within 18 hours from the onset of shock. The study suggested that PCI and coronary artery bypass graft (CABG) were comparable, with similar survival rates at 30 days and 1 year despite more severe and extensive coronary disease in the CABG arm. It is prudent to note that many patients with significant triple vessel disease underwent PCI if the operator opted to based on the severity of shock. There are limited data aside from the SHOCK trial evaluating PCI versus CABG in shock; however, registries continue to report similar outcomes with PCI and CABG with the limitation that CABG is performed in less than 5% of cases of CS.[40]

The decision to perform culprit only versus multivessel PCI has been a topic of ongoing research and controversy. Based on observational studies, the 2017 European and 2013 US guidelines recommended multivessel PCI in AMI-CS. The landmark CULPRIT SHOCK trial (Culprit lesion only PCI vs multi-vessel PCI in Cardiogenic Shock) prospectively randomized revascularization strategy in patients with multivessel coronary artery disease presenting with STEMI and CS. CULPRIT-SHOCK demonstrated a significant absolute reduction in 30-day mortality using a culprit-only revascularization strategy versus an initial strategy of complete revascularization during the index procedure.[41] Despite the CULPRIT-SHOCK trial including the unusual practice of acute chronic total occlusion PCI in an effort to provide complete revascularization during the index procedure, there is physiologic

basis for their finding. Nonculprit PCI can affect short-term outcomes by causing transient cessation of blood flow and microembolization, impairing LV function and hemodynamics.[42] Thus, more extensive multivessel revascularization in patients in CS may lead to transient worsening of LV function and risk of hemodynamic collapse, particularly when performed without MCS.[9] Following the publication of the CULPRIT-SHOCK trial, the 2018 European guidelines updated their recommendations for multivessel disease in CS, with non-infarct-related artery PCI receiving a class III recommendation.

Mechanical Circulatory Support

Numerous devices are available to provide hemodynamic support in CS (Table 2). MCS devices support hemodynamics, augment end-organ perfusion, and limit the need for escalating doses of inotropes and vasopressors. MCS can be used in multiple configurations and combinations to support both univentricular and biventricular shock.

The mechanism of action of intraaortic balloon pump counterpulsation (IABP) is counterpulsation. IABPs inflate during diastole and deflate during systole, resulting in increased coronary blood flow and decreased afterload. IABPs are the most widely studied and used form of MCS. Early evidence on the efficacy of IABP in AMI-CS was based primarily on registry data. The IABP Shock II trial, the first large randomized controlled trial of MCS in AMI-CS,

Table 2
Mechanical circulatory support

	IABP	Impella	Tandem	VA-ECMO
Flow (L/min)	0.5–1	2.5 3.5 5.0 5.5	3.5–4.5	3–6
Mechanism of action	Counterpulsation	Transvalvular microaxial pump	Centrifugal cardiac bypass	Centrifugal cardiopulmonary bypass
Sheath size	7–8F	2.5–13F CP–14F 5.0–23F (cut down) 5.5–19F (cut down)	Inflow: 17F Outflow: 15–19F	Inflow: 21–29F Outflow: 15–19F
Effect on cardiac output	↑	↑↑	↑↑	↑↑
Effect on afterload	→	→	↑	↑↑
Effect on LVEDP	↓	↓↓	↓↓	↕
Effect on Coronary perfusion	↑	↑	↕	↕
Advantages	Simple cannulation, low hemolysis profile, easy to transport patient	Simple cannulation, unloading of the LV, antegrade flow	Indirect unloading of the LV	Biventricular support, oxygenation, simple cannulation
Disadvantages	Requires intrinsic heart function, modest hemodynamic support	Large-bore access, risk of hemolysis	Large-bore access, retrograde blood flow, requires atrial septostomy	Large-bore access, retrograde blood flow

evaluated 30-day mortality in patients with AMI-CS with plans to undergo early revascularization in patients randomized to primary PCI versus primary PCI with up-front IABP insertion.[43] The trial demonstrated no mortality benefit with the routine use of IABP in patients with AMI-CS.[44] Multiple subsequent studies have failed to demonstrate improved outcomes with the use of IABP, and as a result, US and European guidelines both downgraded recommendations for IABP in AMI-CS to class IIB in the United States and a class III in Europe.

The Impella (Abiomed, Danvers, MA) is an axial flow percutaneous ventricular assist device (VAD) that is commercially available in 4 sizes (2.5, CP, 5.0, 5.5) corresponding with the level of LV support as well as the Impella RP, which is a dedicated right-sided support device. Early evidence from the Impella-EUROSHOCK registry evaluated the use of Impella 2.5 in AMI-CS. Despite improved end-organ perfusion as evidenced by reduced lactate levels, the study was unable to show a mortality benefit at 30 days among patients treated with Impella.[45] Similar findings were reported from the USpella registry, which additionally suggested that early use of hemodynamic support is favorable in stabilizing hemodynamics by direct unloading of the left ventricle.[46] These positive trends in the registry data prompted the IMPRESS trial (Impella CP vs Intraaortic balloon pump in Acute Myocardial Infarction Complicated by Cardiogenic Shock). The IMPRESS trial was a multicenter, randomized controlled trial that randomized patients with AMI-CS to Impella CP versus IABP.[47] This trial failed to show mortality benefit for the use of Impella at 30 days or 6 months. The IMPRESS trial is limited by small sample size and low statistical power to detect differences between treatment groups as well as the high level of acuity of patients included in the trial. Of the patients in the IMPRESS trial, 92% suffered cardiac arrest and 48% of those patients had delayed return of spontaneous circulation (ROSC) greater than 20 minutes. Given this very sick cohort, application to patients earlier in the shock cascade may be limited. The IMPRESS trial and 2 other trials were examined in a meta-analysis that showed lower in-hospital mortality and lower 30-day mortality with the use of Impella when implemented pre-PCI versus post-PCI.[48] Single-center data suggest favorable outcomes with the use of Impella 5.0 as a bridge to VAD.[49]

Another available MCS device is the TandemHeart. The TandemHeart (LivaNova, London, UK) is a centrifugal flow pump in which blood is directly withdrawn from the left atrium, indirectly offloading the left ventricle, and propelled into the arterial system via an arterial cannula inserted into the common femoral artery. TandemHeart insertion requires additional expertise in transseptal access to deliver the left atrial cannula. The data on the use of TandemHeart in AMI-CS are limited but suggest that when compared with IABP, there is a trend toward improved hemodynamics, with improvement in renal function and urine output and decrease in lactate. TandemHeart, however, may be associated with more significant vascular complications because of the need for 17- to 19F arterial access.[50]

Extracorporeal membrane oxygenation (ECMO) is cardiopulmonary bypass that can be placed both surgically and percutaneously in the cardiac catheterization laboratory. In the venoarterial configuration, it is increasingly being used as a method to provide maximal hemodynamic support in CS. Registry data from ELSO show that patients with AMI and CS have a high acuity of illness as evidenced by lower arterial pH, blood pressure, and cardiac output as well as a higher proportion of patients postcardiac arrest on mechanical ventilation.[51] Survival to discharge in this group of patients is 40.2%, similar to patients with non-AMI CS. ECMO and temporary circulatory support have been shown to be effective in reversing end-organ dysfunction and stabilizing hemodynamics as a bridge to recovery, VAD, or transplant.[52,53] A recently published retrospective study characterized outcomes of awake patients on VA-ECMO who are supported as a bridge to recovery, VAD, or transplant.[54] The results showed that VA-ECMO resulted in an 83% overall risk reduction in mortality and improved end-organ function comparable to lower-acuity INTERMACs categories.[54] The ECMO data to date are limited to registries for all comers in CS and lack prospective, randomized trials. The ECMO-CS trial is an ongoing European prospective multicenter, randomized controlled trial that will evaluate the safety, efficacy, early, and late mortality benefit of early conservative therapy versus early implantation of VA-ECMO, and it is hoped, will clarify the role of VA-ECMO in patients with CS.[55]

Last, RV failure after MI portends a poor prognosis and is an independent predictor of poor outcomes, including heart failure and death.[56] The devices available that support RV function are the Impella RP and Tandem Protek Duo. The Impella RP is an axial flow pump that provides RV support by pulling blood from the inferior vena cava and expelling it into the PA. The

Tandem Protek Duo is a centrifugal flow pump that pulls blood from the right atrium and propels it into the PA. There are limited data available for use in AMI complicated by CS.

Shock Systems of Care

Given the high mortality associated with AMI-CS, health care systems and clinicians are increasingly using CS systems of care. These systems of care have blossomed because of the following factors. First, recruiting and enrolling patients into CS studies has been difficult. These patients are critically ill and require immediate medical stabilization for which clinicians are reluctant to delay care. Historically, less than 0.025% of patients have been enrolled into randomized controlled trials. The difficulties in conducting high-quality and well-powered trials have led to lack of standardization of care. The utility of simple tools, such as invasive hemodynamics and PA catheters, is practiced variably from hospital to hospital. Data in regard to routine medical interventions, such as antiplatelet therapies and use of inotropes and vasopressors, are similarly scarce. Over the past decade, there has been significant advancement in the availability and use of MCS devices. These devices are smaller and more mobile and have led to the diffuse of shock management. Shock is not managed solely by surgical services and ECMO, but more frequently by interventional, heart failure, and critical care cardiologists with numerous univentricular and biventricular devices.

Shock protocols allow for a uniform treatment strategy in an effort to provide patients, nurses, and clinicians a systematic pathway of care, while shock teams provide a diverse set of options that can be catered to the individual patient, taking into account operator and institutional expertise (Fig. 2). This concept is best exemplified in the work of the National Cardiogenic Shock Initiative. Investigators began by reviewing outcomes data in AMI-CS and forming best practices, which were put together into a shock protocol (see Fig. 2). The study was limited to evaluating outcomes in patients with AMI-CS and not other shock phenotypes. The study also used inclusion and exclusion criteria similar to previous randomized controlled trials in an effort to compare with prior work. A 41-patient pilot study found the protocol could be used across selected centers and was associated with high survival when compared with historical studies and local outcomes.[57] In total, greater than 60 sites were recruited with a goal to enroll 400 patients. The National Cardiogenic Shock Initiative is the first contemporary study to evaluate outcomes of a shock protocol (Fig. 3).[58] The best practices included in the protocol are (1) to identify AMI-CS early and treat patients in the catheterization laboratory (early is defined as <90–120 minutes of diagnosis and before escalating use of

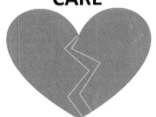

EMERGENCY DEPARTMENT	CARDIOGENIC SHOCK CARE	INTENSIVE CARE UNIT

EMERGENCY DEPARTMENT
Prompt Identification
Early Cath Lab Activation
Hemodynamic Stabilization
Inotropes
• NE>Dopamine
IV Anticoagulation
Antiplatelet Therapy
• Consider IV Agent

CARDIAC CATH LAB
Invasive Hemodynamics
• Uni- vs Bi- Ventricular Failure
MCS (Pre-PCI)
• Meticulous Access (U/S, Fluoro)
• Reperfusion Sheath PRN
Early Revascularization
• Image Guided (IVUS)
• Culprit Only (Selective MV-PCI)
Serial Hemodynamics
• RV Failure? (RA, PAPI, PCWP:RA)
• Escalation (Inotropes, CPO, Lactate)
• Weaning (Inotropes, CPO, PA Sat)

CARDIOGENIC SHOCK CARE

• Care is best delivered based upon local expertise, taking into account operator and institutional strengths, weaknesses and experience.
• A low threshold should be maintained for escalating patient's care to advanced heart failure and transplant centers as soon as such a need is identified

INTENSIVE CARE UNIT
Optimize End Organ Function
• Ventilatory Management
• Dialysis PRN
• Neuro Protection/Hypothermia PRN
Continued Serial Hemodynamics
• RV Failure? (RA, PAPI, PCWP:RA)
• Escalation (Inotropes, CPO, Lactate)
• Weaning (Inotropes, CPO, PA Sat)
Minimize MCS Risk
• Limb Ischemia
• Bleeding/Hemolysis
• CVA
Heart Team
• CTS
• Adv Heart Failure
• Palliative Care

FLOOR/DISCHARGE/REHAB
Life Vest/ICD
Goal Directed Medical Therapy
Close Follow
• Continued High 1-year Mortality

Fig. 2. Team-based management in CS management. PRN, as needed. CPO, cardiac power output; CTS, cardiothoracic surgery; CVA, cerebrovascular accident; ICD, implantable cardioventer-defibrillator; IVUS, intra-vascular ultrasound; NE, norepinephrine; PA Sat, pulmonary artery saturation; U/S, ultrasound.

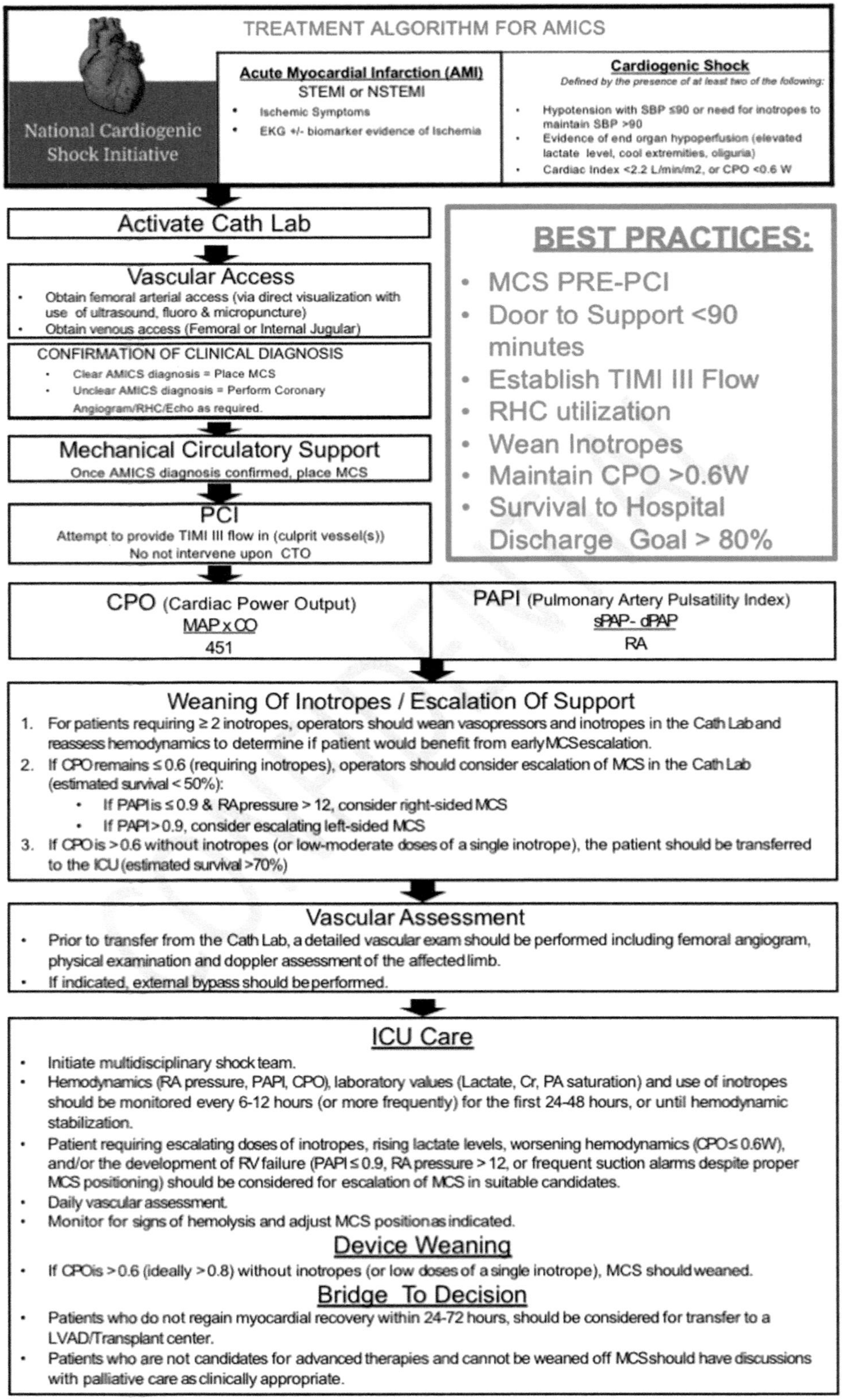

TREATMENT ALGORITHM FOR AMICS

National Cardiogenic Shock Initiative

Acute Myocardial Infarction (AMI)
STEMI or NSTEMI
- Ischemic Symptoms
- EKG +/- biomarker evidence of Ischemia

Cardiogenic Shock
Defined by the presence of at least two of the following:
- Hypotension with SBP ≤90 or need for inotropes to maintain SBP >90
- Evidence of end organ hypoperfusion (elevated lactate level, cool extremities, oliguria)
- Cardiac Index <2.2 L/min/m2, or CPO <0.6 W

Activate Cath Lab

Vascular Access
- Obtain femoral arterial access (via direct visualization with use of ultrasound, fluoro & micropuncture)
- Obtain venous access (Femoral or Internal Jugular)

CONFIRMATION OF CLINICAL DIAGNOSIS
- Clear AMICS diagnosis = Place MCS
- Unclear AMICS diagnosis = Perform Coronary Angiogram/RHC/Echo as required.

Mechanical Circulatory Support
Once AMICS diagnosis confirmed, place MCS

PCI
Attempt to provide TIMI III flow in (culprit vessel(s))
No not intervene upon CTO

BEST PRACTICES:
- MCS PRE-PCI
- Door to Support <90 minutes
- Establish TIMI III Flow
- RHC utilization
- Wean Inotropes
- Maintain CPO >0.6W
- Survival to Hospital Discharge Goal > 80%

CPO (Cardiac Power Output)
$$\frac{MAP \times CO}{451}$$

PAPI (Pulmonary Artery Pulsatility Index)
$$\frac{sPAP - dPAP}{RA}$$

Weaning Of Inotropes / Escalation Of Support
1. For patients requiring ≥ 2 inotropes, operators should wean vasopressors and inotropes in the Cath Lab and reassess hemodynamics to determine if patient would benefit from early MCS escalation.
2. If CPO remains ≤ 0.6 (requiring inotropes), operators should consider escalation of MCS in the Cath Lab (estimated survival < 50%):
   - If PAPI is ≤ 0.9 & RA pressure > 12, consider right-sided MCS
   - If PAPI > 0.9, consider escalating left-sided MCS
3. If CPO is > 0.6 without inotropes (or low-moderate doses of a single inotrope), the patient should be transferred to the ICU (estimated survival >70%)

Vascular Assessment
- Prior to transfer from the Cath Lab, a detailed vascular exam should be performed including femoral angiogram, physical examination and doppler assessment of the affected limb.
- If indicated, external bypass should be performed.

ICU Care
- Initiate multidisciplinary shock team.
- Hemodynamics (RA pressure, PAPI, CPO), laboratory values (Lactate, Cr, PA saturation) and use of inotropes should be monitored every 6-12 hours (or more frequently) for the first 24-48 hours, or until hemodynamic stabilization.
- Patient requiring escalating doses of inotropes, rising lactate levels, worsening hemodynamics (CPO ≤ 0.6W), and/or the development of RV failure (PAPI ≤ 0.9, RA pressure > 12, or frequent suction alarms despite proper MCS positioning) should be considered for escalation of MCS in suitable candidates.
- Daily vascular assessment.
- Monitor for signs of hemolysis and adjust MCS position as indicated.

Device Weaning
- If CPO is > 0.6 (ideally > 0.8) without inotropes (or low doses of a single inotrope), MCS should weaned.

Bridge To Decision
- Patients who do not regain myocardial recovery within 24-72 hours, should be considered for transfer to a LVAD/Transplant center.
- Patients who are not candidates for advanced therapies and cannot be weaned off MCS should have discussions with palliative care as clinically appropriate.

Fig. 3. National CS protocol. EKG, electrocardiogram; ICU, intensive care unit; LVAD, left ventricular assist device; SBP, systolic blood pressure.

inotropes);(2) to place MCS before PCI, as PCI can result in reperfusion injury, distal embolization, and transient cessation of coronary perfusion with balloon inflations and stents, which are better tolerated with MCS; and (3) to use PA catheters to assess patients underlying hemodynamic state and to guide further therapy, including escalation of MCS, identification of RV failure, and weaning. The study has enrolled more than 300 patients with AMI-CS and has demonstrated a survival to hospital discharge rate greater than 70%.[59] Similar improved outcomes have been published by individual health care system as well.[60,61]

SUMMARY

AMI complicated by CS is associated with significant morbidity and mortality. Few therapies have been evaluated in well-powered randomized controlled trials. The use of expert clinicians and formalized shock systems of care is associated with improved outcomes.

DISCLOSURE

M.B. Basir is a consultant for Abbott Vascular, Abiomed, Cardiovascular Systems, Chiesi, Procyrion, and Zoll. All other authors report no conflict of interest.

REFERENCES

1. Hunziker L, Radovanovic D, Jeger R, et al. Twenty-year trends in the incidence and outcome of cardiogenic shock in the AMIS plus registry. Circ Cardiovasc Interv 2019;12:3007293.
2. De Luca L, Olivari Z, Farina A, et al. Temporal trends in the epidemiology, management, and outcome of patients with cardiogenic shock complication acute coronary syndromes: management changes in cardiogenic shock. Eur J Heart Fail 2015;17:1124–32.
3. Kolte D, Khera SM, Aronow WS, et al. Trends in incidence, management, and outcomes of cardiogenic shock complication ST-elevation myocardial infarction in the United States. J Am Heart Assoc 2014;3:e000590.
4. Goldberg RJ, Gore JM, Alpert JS, et al. Cardiogenic shock after acute myocardial infarction: incidence and mortality from a community-wide perspective, 1970 to 1988. N Engl J Med 1991;325:1117–22.
5. Hochman JS, Sleeper LA, White HD, et al. One-year survival following early revascularization for cardiogenic shock. JAMA 2001;285(2):190–2.
6. Hochman JS, Sleeper LA, Webb JG, et al. Early revascularization in acute myocardial infarction complicated by cardiogenic shock. N Engl J Med 1999;341(9):625–34.
7. Harjola VP, Lassus J, Sionis A, et al. Clinical picture and risk prediction of short-term mortality in cardiogenic shock. Eur J Heart Fail 2015;17(5):501–9.
8. Poss J, Koster J, Fuernau G, et al. Risk stratification for patients in cardiogenic shock after acute myocardial infarction. J Am Coll Cardiol 2017;69(15):1913–20.
9. Thiele H, Zeymer U, Neumann FJ, et al. Intraaortic balloon support for myocardial infarction with cardiogenic shock. N Engl J Med 2012;367:1287–96.
10. Vahdatpour C, Collin D, Goldberg S. Cardiogenic shock. J Am Heart Assoc 2019;8:e011991.
11. Baran DA, Grines CL, Bailey S, et al. SCAI clinical expert consensus statement on the classification of cardiogenic shock. Catheter Cardiovasc Interv 2019;94:29–37.
12. Jentzer JC, van Diepen S, Barness GW, et al. Cardiogenic shock classification to predict mortality in the cardiac intensive care unit. J Am Coll Cardiol 2019;74(17):2117–28.
13. Hochman JS. Cardiogenic shock complicating acute myocardial infarction: expanding the paradigm. Circulation 2003;107:2998–3002.
14. Kohsaka S, Menon V, Lowe AM, et al. Systemic inflammatory response syndrome after acute myocardial infarction complicated by cardiogenic shock. Arch Intern Med 2005;165:1643–50.
15. Shah AH, Puri R, Kalra A. Management of cardiogenic shock complicating acute myocardial infarction: a review. Clin Cardiol 2019;42:484–93.
16. Harjola VP, Mebazaa A, Celutkiene J, et al. Contemporary management of acute right ventricular failure: a statement from the Heart Failure Association and the Working Group on Pulmonary Circulation and Right Ventricular Function of the European Society of Cardiology. Eur J Heart Fail 2016;18:226–41.
17. Jacobs AK, Leopold JA, Bates E, et al. Cardiogenic shock caused by right ventricular infarction: a report from the SHOCK registry. Circulation 2003;41:1273–9.
18. Braat SH, Brugada P, deZwaan C, et al. Value of electrocardiogram in diagnosing right ventricular involvement in patients with acute inferior wall myocardial infarction. Br Heart J 1983;49:368–72.
19. Kinch JW, Ryan TJ. Right ventricular infarction. N Engl J Med 1994;330(17):1211–7.
20. Brodie BR, Stuckey TD, Hansen C, et al. Comparison of late survival in patients with cardiogenic shock due to right ventricular infarction versus left ventricular pump failure following primary percutaneous coronary intervention for ST-elevation acute myocardial infarction. Am J Cardiol 2007;99:431–5.
21. Korabathina R, Heffernan KS, Paruchi V, et al. The pulmonary artery pulsatility index identifies severe

right ventricular dysfunction in acute inferior myocardial infarction. Catheter Cardiovasc Interv 2012;80:593–600.

22. Kuchibhotla S, Esposito ML, Breton C, et al. Acute biventricular mechanical circulatory support for cardiogenic shock. J Am Heart Assoc 2017;6(10):e006670.

23. Reynolds HR, Hochman JS. Cardiogenic shock: current concepts and improving outcomes. Circulation 2008;117:686–97.

24. Chen ZM, Pan HC, Chen YP, et al. Early intravenous then oral metoprolol in 45,852 patients with acute myocardial infarction: randomized placebo-controlled trial. Lancet 2005;366(9497):1622–32.

25. Mohammad MA, Andell P, Koul S, et al. Intravenous beta-blocker therapy in ST-segment elevation myocardial infarction treated with primary percutaneous coronary intervention is not associated with benefit regarding short term mortality: a Swedish nationwide observational study. EuroIntervtion 2017;13(2):e210–8.

26. Weeks PA, Sieg A, Paruthi C, et al. Antiplatelet therapy considerations in ischemic cardiogenic shock: implications of metabolic bioactivation. J Cardiovasc Pharm Ther 2015;20(4):370–7.

27. Na SJ, Chung CR, Cho YH, et al. Vasoactive inotropic score as a predictor of mortality in adult patients with cardiogenic shock: medical therapy versus ECMO. Rev Esp Cardiol (Engl E) 2019;72(1):40–7.

28. Werdan K, Gielen S, Ebelt H, et al. Mechanical circulatory support in cardiogenic shock. Eur Heart J 2014;35:156–67.

29. O'Connor CM, Gattis WA, Uretsky BF, et al. Continuous intravenous dobutamine is associated with an increased risk of death in patients with advanced heart failure: insights from the Flolan International Randomized Survival Trial (FIRST). Am Heart J 1999;138:78–86.

30. Abraham WT, Adams KF, Fonarow GC, et al. In-hospital morality in patients with acute decompensated heart failure requiring intravenous vasoactive medications: an analysis from the acute decompensated heart failure national registry (ADHERE). J Am Coll Cardiol 2005;46(1):57–64.

31. Jentzer JC, Coons JC, Link CB, et al. Pharmacotherapy update on the use of vasopressors and inotropes in the intensive care unit. J Cardiovasc Pharm Theapeutics 2015;23(3):249–60.

32. De Backer D, Biston P, Devriendt J, et al. Comparison of dopamine and norepinephrine in the treatment of shock. N Engl J Med 2010;362(9):779–89.

33. Jentzer JC, Wiley B, Bennett C, et al. Temporal trends and clinical outcomes associated with vasopressor and inotrope use in the cardiac intensive care unit. Shock 2020;53(4):452–9.

34. Tarvasmaki T, Lassus J, Varpula M, et al. "Current real-life use of vasopressors and inotropes in cardiogenic shock – adrenaline use is associated with excess organ injury and morality. Crit Care 2016;20(1):208.

35. Leopold V, Gayat E, Pirracchio R, et al. Epinephrine and short-term survival in cardiogenic shock: an individual data meta-analysis of 2583 patients. Intensive Crit Care Med 2018;44(6):847–56.

36. White HD, Van de Werf FJ. Thrombolysis for acute myocardial infarction. Circulation 1998;97(16):1632–46.

37. Zijlstra F, Hoorntje JC, de Boer MJ, et al. Long-term benefit of primary angioplasty as compared with thrombolytic therapy for acute myocardial infarction. N Engl J Med 1999;341(19):1413–9.

38. Hasdai D, Califf RM, Thompson TD, et al. Predictors of cardiogenic shock after thrombolytic therapy for acute myocardial infarction. J Am Coll Cardiol 2000;35(1):136–43.

39. Hochman JS, Buller CE, Sleeper LA, et al. Cardiogenic shock complicating acute myocardial infarction–etiologies, management and outcome: a report from the SHOCK Trial Registry. SHould we emergently revascularize Occluded Coronaries for cardiogenic shocK? J Am Coll Cardiol 2000;36(3 Suppl A):1063–70.

40. White HD, Assmann SF, Sanborn TA, et al. Comparison of percutaneous coronary intervention and coronary artery bypass grafting after acute myocardial infarction complicated by cardiogenic shock: results from the Should We Emergently Revascularize Occluded Coronaries for Cardiogenic Shock (SHOCK) trial. Circulation 2005;112(13):1992–2001.

41. Thiele H, Desch S. CULPRIT-SHOCK (Culprit Lesion Only PCI Versus Multivessel Percutaneous Coronary Intervention in Cardiogenic Shock): implications on guideline recommendations. Circulation 2018;137(13):1314–6.

42. Brener M, Rosenblum H, Basir M, et al. Hemodynamics of high-risk percutaneous coronary intervention with and without mechanical circulatory support: a pilot study with pressure volume loop analysis. J Am Coll Cardiol 2019;74(13 Supplement):B316.

43. Thiele H, Schuler G, Neumann FJ, et al. Intraaortic balloon pump in cardiogenic shock complicating acute myocardial infarction: long-term 6-year outcome of the randomized IABP-SHOCK II trial. Circulation 2018.

44. Unverzagt S, Buerke M, de Waha A, et al. Intra-aortic balloon pump counterpulsation (IABP) for myocardial infarction complicated by cardiogenic shock. Cochrane Database Syst Rev 2015;(3):CD007398.

45. Lauten A, Engstrom AE, Jung C, et al. Percutaneous left-ventricular support with the Impella-2.5-assist device in acute cardiogenic shock: results

of the Impella-EUROSHOCK-registry. Circ Heart Fail 2013;6(1):23–30.

46. O'Neill WW, Schreiber T, Wohns DH, et al. The current use of Impella 2.5 in acute myocardial infarction complicated by cardiogenic shock: results from the USpella Registry. J Interv Cardiol 2014; 27(1):1–11.

47. Ouweneel DM, Erikson E, Sjauw KD, et al. Impella CP versus intraaortic balloon pump in acute myocardial infarction complicated by cardiogenic shock. JACC 2016.

48. Flaherty MP, Khan AR, O'Neill WW. Early initiation of Impella in acute myocardial infarction complicated by cardiogenic shock improves survival: a meta-analysis. JACC Cardiovasc Interv 2017; 10(17):1805–6.

49. Lima B, Kale P, Gonzalez-Stawinski GV, et al. Effectiveness and Safety of the Impella 5.0 as a Bridge to Cardiac Transplantation or Durable Left Ventricular Assist Device. Am J Cardiol 2016;117(10):1622–8. https://doi.org/10.1016/j.amjcard.2016.02.038.

50. Thiele H, Sick P, Boudriot E, et al. Randomized comparison of intra-aortic balloon support with a percutaneous left ventricular assist device in patients with revascularized acute myocardial infarction complicated by cardiogenic shock. Eur Heart J 2005; 26(13):1276–83.

51. Acharya D, Torabi M, Borgstrom M, et al. Extracorporeal membrane oxygenation in myocardial infarction complicated by cardiogenic shock: analysis of the ELSO Registry. J Am Coll Cardiol 2020; 76(8):1001–2.

52. Rousse N, Juthier F, Pincon C, et al. ECMO as a bridge to decision: recovery, VAD, or heart transplantation? Int J Cardiol 2015;187:620–7.

53. Shah P, Pagani FD, Desai SS, et al. Outcomes of patients receiving temporary circulatory support before durable ventricular assist device. Ann Thorac Surg 2017;103(1):106–12.

54. Mori M, McCloskey G, Geirsson A, et al. Improving outcomes in INTERMACS category 1 patients with pre-LVAD, awake venous-arterial extracorporeal membrane oxygenation support. ASAIO J 2019; 65(8):819–26.

55. Ostadal P, Rokyta R, Kruger A, et al. Extra corporeal membrane oxygenation in the therapy of cardiogenic shock (ECMO-CS): rationale and design of the multicenter randomized trial. Eur J Heart Fail 2017;19(Suppl 2):124–7.

56. Zornoff LA, Skali H, Pfeffer MA, et al. Right ventricular dysfunction and risk of heart failure and mortality after myocardial infarction. J Am Coll Cardiol 2002;39(9):1450–5.

57. Basir MB, Schreiber T, Dixon S, et al. Feasibility of early mechanical circulatory support in acute myocardial infarction complicated by cardiogenic shock: the Detroit Cardiogenic Shock Initiative. Catheter Cardiovasc Interv 2018;91(3):454–61.

58. Basir MB, Kapur NK, Patel K, et al, National Cardiogenic Shock Initiative Investigators. Improved outcomes associated with the use of shock protocols: updates from the national cardiogenic shock initiative. Catheter Cardiovasc Interv 2019;93(7):1173–83.

59. Lemor A, Basir MB, Patel K, et al, National Cardiogenic Shock Initiative Investigators. Multivessel versus culprit-vessel percutaneous coronary intervention in cardiogenic shock. JACC Cardiovasc Interv 2020;13(10):1171–8.

60. Tehrani BN, Truesdell AG, Sherwood MW, et al. Standardized team-based care for cardiogenic shock. J Am Coll Cardiol 2019;73(13):1659–69. Erratum in: J Am Coll Cardiol. 2019 Jul 23;74(3): 481. PMID: 30947919.

61. Taleb I, Koliopoulou AG, Tandar A, et al. Shock team approach in refractory cardiogenic shock requiring short-term mechanical circulatory support: a proof of concept. Circulation 2019;140(1):98–100.

ST-Elevation Myocardial Infarction Complicated by Out-of-Hospital Cardiac Arrest

Marinos Kosmopoulos, MD, Jason A. Bartos, MD, PhD,
Demetris Yannopoulos, MD*

KEYWORDS

- Cardiac arrest • ST-Elevation myocardial infarction • Acute coronary syndrome • Hypothermia
- Antiplatelet

KEY POINTS

- Patients with myocardial infarction with ST elevation have worse outcomes in case of an out-of-hospital cardiac arrest.
- Coronary angiography is frequently omitted or delayed in patients with cardiac arrest with ST elevation despite the survival benefit it yields.
- ST-elevation myocardial infarctions have higher risk for in-stent thrombosis in patients with out-of-hospital cardiac arrest. Ticagrelor and prasugrel are the antiplatelets of choice for combination with aspirin in dual antiplatelet therapy.
- Therapeutic hypothermia can be safely applied in revascularized patients with out-of-hospital cardiac arrest.
- Successfully revascularized patients with cardiac arrest surviving to hospital discharge do not yield any additional long-term survival benefit from the implantation of cardiac defibrillators.

INTRODUCTION

Approximately 350,000 patients suffered an out-of-hospital cardiac arrest (OHCA) in 2015 (Fig. 1). Among those who survive to hospital admission, only 10.4% survived to discharge.[1] Cardiac arrest can be further classified as refractory, depending on whether the patient achieves and maintains return of spontaneous circulation (ROSC) or not. For resuscitated patients presenting with initial shockable rhythms, mortality has been estimated at 55% to 70%.[2–4] More than 1,000,000 hospitalizations every year are due to an acute coronary syndrome (ACS),[1] with an in-hospital mortality of myocardial infarction (MI) approximately 2.5% to 7.4%.[1,5]

Although ACS and cardiac arrest are separate clinical entities, they are strongly linked. Approximately 5% to 10% of ST-elevation MIs (STEMIs) present with OHCA.[6,7] Clinically significant coronary artery disease (CAD) has also been reported in 30% to 45% of patients presenting with resuscitated ventricular tachycardia/ventricular fibrillation (VT/VF) OHCA without ST elevation, 70% to 90% of patients with resuscitated VT/VF OHCA with ST elevation, and in 55% to 85% of patients with refractory shockable cardiac arrest treated with extracorporeal membrane oxygenation cardiopulmonary resuscitation (eCPR).[8–13] Moreover, autopsy studies suggest that up to 80% of people who died from OHCA were found to have high-grade coronary artery stenosis as the underlying cause.[14,15] Controversy exists regarding the interventional strategies for the optimal management of these patients, as the need to

Cardiovascular Division, Center for Resuscitation Medicine, University of Minnesota Medical School, University of Minnesota, 420 Delaware Street SE, Minneapolis, MN 55455, USA
* Corresponding author. Center for Resuscitation Medicine, University of Minnesota Medical School, 420 Delaware Street SE, MMC 508 Mayo, Minneapolis, MN 55401.
E-mail address: yanno001@umn.edu

Intervent Cardiol Clin 10 (2021) 359–368
https://doi.org/10.1016/j.iccl.2021.03.007
2211-7458/21/© 2021 Elsevier Inc. All rights reserved.

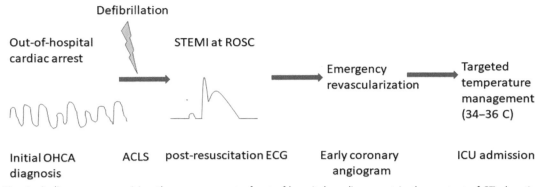

Fig. 1. A diagram summarizing the management of out-of-hospital cardiac arrest in the context of ST elevation myocardial infarction. ACLS, advanced cardiovascular life support; ICU, intensive care unit.

improve outcomes remains. Patients with OHCA STEMI are a unique cardiac arrest population, as they are the most likely to have a reversible cause for OHCA and can significantly benefit from the correct and rapid application of therapeutic strategies.[16] However, they have been excluded from most randomized clinical trials examining revascularization in the setting of ACS and their outcomes are not disclosed in public reports.[17] Thus, uncertainty exists regarding the applicability and efficacy of the recent therapeutic advances on this high-risk STEMI population. This review summarizes and presents the literature evidence for the best management of patients with STEMI in the context of cardiac arrest.

GUIDELINE RECOMMENDATIONS

Despite the sparsity of clinical data, there are specific recommendations for the management of OHCA. Both the American Heart Association and the European Society of Cardiology recommend primary percutaneous coronary intervention (PCI) in all patients with resuscitated OHCA and evidence of STEMI,[18,19] whereas a lower degree of indication (IIa) is recommended for patients with suspicion of MI and not ST elevation.[19] The European Society of Cardiology also proposes the application of therapeutic hypothermia for the first 24 hours of hospitalization.[19]

FIELD MANAGEMENT AND EARLY CORONARY ANGIOGRAPHY

ST segment elevation in the initial electrocardiogram (ECG) after successful resuscitation of OHCA is associated with the presence of a culprit lesion, and revascularization should always be (if possible) attempted.[20] Over the past decade, patient admission to PCI-capable centers has

increased substantially, and this strategy has resulted in universal improvement of outcomes.[21–23] However, angiography and revascularization rates are still low in many locations, and additional policy changes might be needed to promote this beneficial care.[24,25] Prehospital emergency medical services can reliably identify STEMI in the post-ROSC electrocardiogram and therefore, activation of the cardiac catheterization laboratory (CCL) should not be delayed.[26] However, it has been noted that only 54% of patients with OHCA MI present with ST elevation and, thus, the absence of ST elevation should not itself preclude a patient from CCL admission.[27] Identification of left bundle branch block and ST depression further improves ECG sensitivity.[23] Chest pain before the arrest is a good predictor of potential MI and should also be taken into consideration.[28] For successfully resuscitated cardiac arrest, hospital volume does not seem to affect the outcomes of patients with OHCA STEMI.[29] Troponin at admission has moderate diagnostic value with a sensitivity of 72% and specificity of 75%, but together with the ECG are reported to detect MI with a 93% sensitivity when a cutoff value of 2.5 ng/mL is applied. Specificity, however, decreases to 64%.[30] Importantly, troponin levels at emergency department admission alone do not offer any reliable information regarding the potential need for revascularization.[31]

Rapid transfer to a PCI-capable center is paramount for the survival of patients with OHCA STEMI. Door-to-balloon time has been reported to range from 39 to 114 minutes.[13,20,32–37] Despite the more critical state of patients with OHCA STEMI, door-to-balloon time is increased compared with their peers presenting without OHCA.[34] Patients with OHCA STEMI tend to have advanced CAD with multiple lesions. Moreover, patients with OHCA STEMI have been noted to have a higher prevalence of chronic totally occluded lesions and this has also been associated with adverse clinical outcomes, especially when its territory is dependent on collateral blood flow from the infarct-related artery.[38] No difference in outcomes has been noted in patients who suffered STEMI complicated by OHCA and had revascularization only in the culprit lesion versus those who underwent multivessel revascularization.[39]

Although its role is undisputed, revascularization with PCI does not come without risks in patients with OHCA STEMI. An observational study reported increased risk of both major bleeding[40] and in-stent thrombosis for patients with OHCA STEMI.[16] The altered pharmacokinetics of antiplatelet agents together with the frequently present hypoxia and metabolic acidosis might drive the incidence of these complications. Moreover, a higher risk of rearrest during revascularization has been observed.[20]

Reports suggest that platelet activity is increased rather than decreased in patients with OHCA of presumed cardiac etiology.[41,42] Antiplatelet therapy should not be delayed, and most revascularized patients with OHCA STEMI still receive dual antiplatelet therapy very early in their management. The selection of therapeutic agents, however, may be challenging. Of all the available agents, ticagrelor seems to be associated with the best outcomes, and both prasugrel and ticagrelor are significantly better than clopidogrel.[43,44] However, there is no randomized trial to solidify these findings. In the Ticagrelor or Prasugrel in Patients with Acute Coronary Syndromes study, the prasugrel group was reported to have a lower incidence of the composite endpoint of death, MI, or stroke; however, no subgroup analysis was available related to patients with cardiac arrest.[45] Moreover, a prospective pharmacokinetic study reported altered bioavailability of ticagrelor in the context of hypothermia. Therefore, dose adjustment might be frequently needed.[46] In case of a comatose patient, ticagrelor can be administered through the nasogastric tube without loss of the therapeutic benefits.[47] Another option may be the use of Cangrelor, which, due to its intravenous administration, avoids concerns regarding unpredictable absorption.[48,49] In general, in sicker patients and especially those presenting with shock, intravenous delivery of the second antiplatelet agent may be a reasonable choice.

REVASCULARIZATION STRATEGIES

Coronary angiography together with PCI is the preferred revascularization method for the emergency treatment of OHCA STEMI.[13,20,32–35,37–39]

There is absence of evidence with regard to the preferred type of stent or the use of percutaneous ventricular assist devices during revascularization.[50] Coronary artery bypass grafting (CABG) is the preferred revascularization strategy for patients with multivessel CAD and diabetes mellitus. Its role in OHCA STEMI management is not clear. A center in Germany reported 79% neurologically intact survival in patients with OHCA STEMI who were treated with CABG in the first 4 hours after admission.[51] CABG is rarely part of the early management of OHCA STEMI in the United States and is reserved only for neurologically intact patients.

ARREST OR REARREST IN THE CARDIAC CATHETERIZATION LABORATORY

Cardiac arrest is infrequent in the CCL, complicating approximately 1% to 6% of all the attempted coronary angiograms and interventions. Cardiac arrest is associated with the severity of the indication and increases in urgent procedures.[52–54] In case of an arrest in the CCL, the best available strategy is the continuation of revascularization while cardiopulmonary resuscitation (CPR) is provided. Mechanical CPR has been associated with superior outcomes compared with manual CPR, and is much safer to the provider, especially given the radiation exposure. Revascularization can be successful in more than 80% of the cases; however, survival is considerably worse compared with the 25.0% to 72.5% mortality that has been reported in patients with OHCA STEMI (Table 1), with a mortality rate between 74.5% and 89.0%.[55–57] An alternative method for successful completion of the procedure might be the application of mechanical support devices, especially percutaneous left ventricular assist devices and veno-arterial extracorporeal membrane oxygenation.[58,59]

NONSHOCKABLE RHYTHMS

Of all cardiac arrests, VF/pulseless VT occurs in only 25%.[1] Most of the studies for OHCA STEMI included patients resuscitated after VF OHCA; however, MI is frequently the cause for VF/VT that is refractory to defibrillation, as well as for pulseless electrical activity and asystole.[60] The Minnesota Resuscitation Consortium has reported that more than 60% of refractory VT/VF is attributed to an ACS.[12] Application of mechanical support through veno-arterial extracorporeal cardiopulmonary membrane oxygenation can provide a bridge to the CCL for these patients.[9,12,61–63] Resuscitated nonshockable rhythms are considerably less likely to receive coronary angiography

Table 1
Differences between patients suffering from ST-elevation myocardial infarction with and without cardiac arrest

Parameter	OHCA STEMI	STEMI without OHCA
Mean/Median age, y	49.5–68	56.9–68
In-hospital mortality	17.3%–82%	1%–6%
Long-term mortality	25.5%–72.5%	3.5%–26%
Door-to-balloon-time (in minutes)	39–114	36–107
ST-elevation sensitivity/ positive predictive value	60%–98%	94%–98%
% patients treated with angiography median (range)	89% (37%–100%)	93.4% (92.8%–96.4%)
% patients treated with PCI	39.5%–95.6%[6,8,12,16,19,20,22–25,27–30,34,35,42,60–62,68–71,78–80,83–89,91,92]	78.8%–91%
In-stent thrombosis	1.5%–12.3%[16,19,20,56–59,79,80]	0.3%–3.1%

Differences in management and outcomes of patients with ST-elevated myocardial infarction complicated by out-of-hospital cardiac arrest as compared with their non-arrested peers. There is notable variability in the access to reperfusion therapies, that together with the diagnostic challenges and the cerebral injury results in worse short-term and long-term survival.

Abbreviations: OHCA, out-of-hospital cardiac arrest; PCI, percutaneous coronary intervention; STEMI, ST-elevated myocardial infarction.

compared with patients with OHCA VT/VF,[34,60,64,65] but the incidence of ACS remains unknown. Even for those who receive coronary angiography, survival is significantly lower for patients with nonshockable rhythms compared with those with shockable rhythms with STEMI and patients with STEMI without cardiac arrest.[66]

POST PERCUTANEOUS CORONARY INTERVENTION IN-HOSPITAL MANAGEMENT

Consideration of the cause of cardiac arrest and the cause of death in patients with OHCA STEMI presents a paradox. Although the shockable rhythm is triggered by ischemic heart disease in most patients with OHCA STEMI, the most common cause of death is neurologic injury resulting from the cerebral hypoxia during the no-flow and low-flow time of the arrest and resuscitation.[67,68] There is a well-established inverse relationship between time to ROSC and survival that is observed in longitudinal and prospective studies. Thus, both brain recovery and successful myocardial reperfusion are necessary to yield a meaningful survival benefit in patients with STEMI presenting with OHCA.

A major determinant of the patient's treatment course is the level of consciousness before the intervention. Patients who have regained consciousness at the time of CCL admission have excellent outcomes, and their management resembles that of conventional patients with STEMI with short cardiac care unit stay and early hospital discharge.[69] The time course shifts in the cases of comatose patients. Patients are admitted to the intensive care unit, and an extended length of stay is likely, with an average length of stay of 8 days.[25] Compared with successfully resuscitated arrest without ST-elevation, patients with OHCA STEMI are more likely to be unconscious at the time of revascularization,[20] and present with higher creatinine levels.[25] The Global Registry of Acute Coronary Events (GRACE) score has been used to assist with prediction of in-hospital mortality and neurologic outcomes with an area under the receiver-operating characteristic curve of 0.79.[70]

Implantable cardioverter defibrillators are one of the few available tools for secondary prevention of sudden cardiac death and are commonly placed in cardiac arrest survivors. There is significant variability in the rates of implantable cardiac defibrillator implantation around different parts of the world.[71] However, their benefit seems to be limited for patients with STEMI.[72] Neurologic recovery is considerably delayed in patients with OHCA,[10,67] and thus cardiac rehabilitation capacity is significantly lowered in patients with STEMI OHCA with residual cognitive impairment.[73] Nevertheless, patients with OHCA STEMI are noted to have significant improvement in their exercise capacity after 6 weeks of cardiac rehabilitation.[74] There does not seem to be a difference in stress and anxiety levels following the event between OHCA and ambulatory STEMI patients.[75,76]

TARGETED TEMPERATURE MANAGEMENT

Therapeutic hypothermia is commonly applied, although its benefit has been challenged. The randomized clinical trials for hypothermia do not provide subgroup-specific outcomes for patients with STEMI, and therefore conclusions can be inferred only from the general OHCA population. Empirical data tend to favor hypothermia, claiming an improvement in long-term neurologic outcomes,[72] despite the evidence showing that patients treated with hypothermia outside of randomized clinical trials have a higher baseline risk.[77] A clinical trial published in 2017, demonstrated a further improvement in outcomes of patients treated with the combination of hypothermia and Xenon.[78] The published literature supports that hypothermia can be safely applied in revascularized patients with OHCA,[79] as no impairment in coagulation or hypothermia-attributed increase in bleeding and in-stent thrombosis has been noted.[80,81]

The neurologic prognostication of patients who are hospitalized for cardiac arrest remains challenging. Although strategies assessing functional activity of the brain underestimate its recovery, biomarker-based strategies that attempt to quantify neuronal injury rather than brain function holds promise.[68,82] Brain imaging is a definitive marker of brain injury with very high specificity but low sensitivity.[83–85] It is important to remember that neuroprognostication should not be attempted earlier than 72 hours after ROSC. Tight glucose regulation may be necessary, as increased variability in its values is adversely associated with outcomes of patients with OHCA with a cardiac etiology.[86]

LONG-TERM OUTCOMES

Patients with OHCA represent the STEMI population with the highest in-hospital mortality. The reported in-hospital mortality varies considerably. A multicenter study in the United Kingdom documented a center-specific mortality that ranged from 10.7% to 66.3%. Of all the determinants of survival, time to reperfusion emerged as the most robust intervention to improve outcomes.[87]

Because of the exclusion of patients with STEMI OHCA from most randomized clinical trials, there is paucity of data regarding their long-term outcomes and the posthospitalization management. In an OHCA cohort, 1-year mortality of patients with ACS was reported to be 47.1%, with only 37.3% in-hospital mortality. The 18.5% mortality in successfully discharged patients with STEMI is higher than any of the reported mortalities in clinical trials and suggests an increased frailty of patients with STEMI. The patients who died after discharge had multivessel CAD, tended to be significantly older, and had significantly higher prevalence of diabetes mellitus.[88] Cardiac arrest at admission

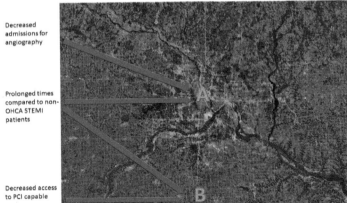

Decreased admissions for angiography

Prolonged times compared to non-OHCA STEMI patients

Decreased access to PCI capable centers

Fig. 2. The yet unmet challenges in STEMI complicated by cardiac arrest in (A) urban and (B) rural settings. Patients with OHCA STEMI in the urban metropolitan areas are underadmitted for angiography compared with their peers without OHCA. In the rural setting, PCI-capable centers are scarce, and in most cases these patients are excluded from regional STEMI networks. In both urban and rural settings, door-to-balloon and symptom-to-balloon times are increased compared with other STEMI populations.

was significantly associated with the 2-year survival of patients with MI, 51% of whom had STEMI.[89] Five-year survival has been reported to be approximately 74.5%,[90] and the same survival was noted for a cohort of patients with OHCA and MI, including 77% of patients with STEMI, who were prospectively followed for 11 years.[25] In a prospective study, the 8-year survival of patients with OHCA STEMI was reported to be 49%, and 78% among the patients who survived to hospital discharge. However, outcomes after discharge did not appear to differ between patients with OHCA STEMI and ambulatory patients with STEMI,[91] This finding is consistent with a report assessing 49,000 patients with STEMI that also did not document any difference in long-term outcomes of patients who survived index hospitalization.[35] Thus, it may be inferred that in-hospital deaths are the main driver for the differences in mortality between patients with OHCA STEMI and ambulatory patients with STEMI.[36]

LIMITATIONS IN TREATMENT ACCESS

A major limitation in the improvement of outcomes of patients with OHCA STEMI is the availability of PCI-capable centers (Fig. 2). It has been documented that for OHCA, the location of the event, the distance from a PCI-capable center, and the reduced population density or a rural location of the arrest are associated with significantly worse outcomes.[21,92] First medical contact-to-device time is reported to be increased for patients with OHCA STEMI in regional systems, implicating it as an important target for improvement of outcomes.[37] Establishment of a regional network for acute care might be a reasonable step toward improvement of outcomes.[21,93] Unfortunately, patients with OHCA are still frequently excluded from regional networks of acute care for STEMI. Access for patients with OHCA STEMI to acute treatment remains largely unaddressed.[94]

Early thrombolysis in OHCA STEMI has also been tested as a potential strategy to improve outcomes for patients with no access to a PCI-capable center. Despite promising case reports,[95] the evidence from practice supports a very limited role of thrombolysis in patients with OHCA STEMI, as it increases major bleeding events without any concomitant improvement in patient outcomes.[95,96] Increased access to PCI-capable centers and creation of networks in the nonurban areas appear to be the most important strategies to improve survival.

SUMMARY

Patients with OHCA STEMI represent a high-mortality population. Rapid coronary angiography can substantially improve outcomes and is associated with lack of residual disability and long-term complications following hospital discharge. Increased risk of in-stent thrombosis, application of therapeutic hypothermia, and selection and monitoring of antiplatelet agents are the greatest challenges for the treating interventional cardiologist.

CLINICS CARE POINTS

- Neuroprognostication of unconscious OHCA STEMI should take place at least 72 hours after the hospitalization.
- The long-term outcomes of OHCA STEMI patients that survive the index hospitalization are comparable to the ambulatory STEMI population.
- The ST-elevation sensitivity is markedly lower in myocardial infarction patients who also suffer from OHCA.
- Mechanical CPR should be the preferred resuscitation approach for an arrest complicating an intervention in the CCL.

DISCLOSURE

The authors have nothing to disclose.

REFERENCES

1. Virani SS, Alonso A, Benjamin EJ, et al. Heart disease and stroke statistics-2020 update: a report From the American Heart Association. Circulation 2020;141(9):e139–596.
2. Hasegawa M, Abe T, Nagata T, et al. The number of prehospital defibrillation shocks and 1-month survival in patients with out-of-hospital cardiac arrest. Scand J Trauma Resusc Emerg Med 2015;23:34.
3. Reynolds JC, Grunau BE, Rittenberger JC, et al. Association between duration of resuscitation and favorable outcome after out-of-hospital cardiac arrest: implications for prolonging or terminating resuscitation. Circulation 2016;134(25):2084–94.
4. Gregers E, Kjaergaard J, Lippert F, et al. Refractory out-of-hospital cardiac arrest with ongoing cardiopulmonary resuscitation at hospital arrival - survival and neurological outcome without extracorporeal cardiopulmonary resuscitation. Crit Care 2018; 22(1):242.

5. Smilowitz NR, Mahajan AM, Roe MT, et al. Mortality of myocardial infarction by sex, age, and obstructive coronary artery disease status in the ACTION Registry-GWTG (Acute Coronary Treatment and Intervention Outcomes Network Registry-Get With the Guidelines). Circ Cardiovasc Qual Outcomes 2017;10(12):e003443.

6. Karam N, Bataille S, Marijon E, et al. Incidence, mortality, and outcome-predictors of sudden cardiac arrest complicating myocardial infarction prior to hospital admission. Circ Cardiovasc Interv 2019; 12(1):e007081.

7. Jabbari R, Engstrøm T, Glinge C, et al. Incidence and risk factors of ventricular fibrillation before primary angioplasty in patients with first ST-elevation myocardial infarction: a nationwide study in Denmark. J Am Heart Assoc 2015;4(1):e001399.

8. Lamhaut L, Tea V, Raphalen JH, et al. Coronary lesions in refractory out of hospital cardiac arrest (OHCA) treated by extra corporeal pulmonary resuscitation (ECPR). Resuscitation 2018;126:154–9.

9. Yannopoulos D, Bartos JA, Aufderheide TP, et al. The evolving role of the cardiac catheterization laboratory in the management of patients with out-of-hospital cardiac arrest: a scientific statement from the American Heart Association. Circulation 2019. https://doi.org/10.1161/CIR.0000000000000630.

10. Bartos JA, Grunau B, Carlson C, et al. Improved survival with extracorporeal cardiopulmonary resuscitation despite progressive metabolic derangement associated with prolonged resuscitation. Circulation 2020;119:042173.

11. Sonneville R, Schmidt M. Extracorporeal cardiopulmonary resuscitation for adults with refractory out-of-hospital cardiac arrest: towards better neurological outcomes. Circulation 2020;141(11):887–90.

12. Yannopoulos D, Bartos JA, Raveendran G, et al. Coronary artery disease in patients with out-of-hospital refractory ventricular fibrillation cardiac arrest. J Am Coll Cardiol 2017;70(9):1109–17.

13. Duerschmied D, Zotzmann V, Rieder M, et al. Myocardial infarction type 1 is frequent in refractory out-of-hospital cardiac arrest (OHCA) treated with extracorporeal cardiopulmonary resuscitation (ECPR). Sci Rep 2020;10(1):8423.

14. Adabag AS, Peterson G, Apple FS, et al. Etiology of sudden death in the community: results of anatomical, metabolic, and genetic evaluation. Am Heart J 2010;159(1):33–9.

15. Davies MJ, Thomas A. Thrombosis and acute coronary-artery lesions in sudden cardiac ischemic death. N Engl J Med 1984;310(18):1137–40.

16. Picard F, Llitjos J-F, Diefenbronn M, et al. The balance of thrombosis and hemorrhage in STEMI patients with or without associated cardiac arrest: An observational study. Resuscitation 2019;145: 83–90.

17. New York State Department of Health. Percutaneous coronary intervention (PCI) in New York state 2010–2012. Albany (NY): New York State Department of Health; 2015. p. 1–74. Available at: https://www.health.ny.gov/statistics/diseases/cardiovascular/docs/pci_2010-2012.pdf.

18. O'Gara PT, Kushner FG, Ascheim DD, et al. 2013 ACCF/AHA guideline for the management of ST-elevation myocardial infarction: a report of the American College of Cardiology Foundation/American Heart Association Task Force on Practice Guidelines. Circulation 2013;127(4):e362–425.

19. Ibanez B, James S, Agewall S, et al. 2017 ESC Guidelines for the management of acute myocardial infarction in patients presenting with ST-segment elevation: The Task Force for the management of acute myocardial infarction in patients presenting with ST-segment elevation of the European Socie. Eur Heart J 2018;39(2):119–77.

20. Kern KB, Lotun K, Patel N, et al. Outcomes of comatose cardiac arrest survivors with and without ST-segment elevation myocardial infarction: importance of coronary angiography. JACC Cardiovasc Interv 2015;8(8):1031–40.

21. Tranberg T, Lippert FK, Christensen EF, et al. Distance to invasive heart centre, performance of acute coronary angiography, and angioplasty and associated outcome in out-of-hospital cardiac arrest: a nationwide study. Eur Heart J 2017;38(21): 1645–52.

22. Shin J, Ko E, Cha WC, et al. Impact of early coronary angiography on the survival to discharge after out-of-hospital cardiac arrest. Clin Exp Emerg Med 2017;4(2):65–72.

23. Sideris G, Voicu S, Dillinger JG, et al. Value of post-resuscitation electrocardiogram in the diagnosis of acute myocardial infarction in out-of-hospital cardiac arrest patients. Resuscitation 2011;82(9):1148–53.

24. Strom JB, McCabe JM, Waldo SW, et al. Management of patients with cardiac arrest complicating myocardial infarction in New York before and after public reporting policy changes. Circ Cardiovasc Interv 2017;10(5). https://doi.org/10.1161/CIRCINTERVENTIONS.116.004833.

25. DeFilippis EM, Singh A, Gupta A, et al. Long-term outcomes after out-of-hospital cardiac arrest in young patients with myocardial infarction. Circulation 2018;138(24):2855–7.

26. Tanguay A, Lebon J, Brassard E, et al. Diagnostic accuracy of prehospital electrocardiograms interpreted remotely by emergency physicians in myocardial infarction patients. Am J Emerg Med 2019;37(7):1242–7.

27. Salam I, Hassager C, Thomsen JH, et al. Editor's Choice—Is the pre-hospital ECG after out-of-hospital cardiac arrest accurate for the diagnosis

of ST-elevation myocardial infarction? Eur Heart J Acute Cardiovasc Care 2016;5(4):317–26.

28. Zeyons F, Jesel L, Morel O, et al. Out-of-hospital cardiac arrest survivors sent for emergency angiography: a clinical score for predicting acute myocardial infarction. Eur Heart J Acute Cardiovasc Care 2017;6(2):103–11.

29. Kontos MC, Fordyce CB, Chen AY, et al. Association of acute myocardial infarction cardiac arrest patient volume and in-hospital mortality in the United States: insights from the national cardiovascular data registry acute coronary treatment and intervention outcomes network registry. Clin Cardiol 2019;42(3):352–7.

30. Voicu S, Sideris G, Deye N, et al. Role of cardiac troponin in the diagnosis of acute myocardial infarction in comatose patients resuscitated from out-of-hospital cardiac arrest. Resuscitation 2012; 83(4):452–8.

31. Pearson DA, Wares CM, Mayer KA, et al. Troponin marker for acute coronary occlusion and patient outcome following cardiac arrest. West J Emerg Med 2015;16(7):1007–13.

32. Maze R, Le May MR, Hibbert B, et al. The impact of therapeutic hypothermia as adjunctive therapy in a regional primary PCI program. Resuscitation 2013; 84(4):460–4.

33. Bro-Jeppesen J, Kjaergaard J, Wanscher M, et al. Emergency coronary angiography in comatose cardiac arrest patients: do real-life experiences support the guidelines? Eur Hear J Acute Cardiovasc Care 2012;1(4):291–301.

34. Velders MA, van Boven N, Boden H, et al. Association between angiographic culprit lesion and out-of-hospital cardiac arrest in ST-elevation myocardial infarction patients. Resuscitation 2013;84(11):1530–5.

35. Alahmar AE, Nelson CP, Snell KIE, et al. Resuscitated cardiac arrest and prognosis following myocardial infarction. Heart 2014;100(14):1125–32.

36. Lee KH, Jeong MH, YoungkeunAhn, et al. One-year clinical impact of cardiac arrest in patients with first onset acute ST-segment elevation myocardial infarction. Int J Cardiol 2014;175(1):147–53.

37. Shavelle DM, Bosson N, Thomas JL, et al. Outcomes of ST elevation myocardial infarction complicated by out-of-hospital cardiac arrest (from the los angeles county regional system). Am J Cardiol 2017;120(5):729–33.

38. Shinouchi K, Ueda Y, Kato T, et al. Relation of chronic total occlusion to in-hospital mortality in the patients with sudden cardiac arrest due to acute coronary syndrome. Am J Cardiol 2019; 123(12):1915–20.

39. Jaguszewski M, Radovanovic D, Nallamothu BK, et al. Multivessel versus culprit vessel percutaneous coronary intervention in ST-elevation myocardial infarction: is more worse? EuroIntervention 2013; 9(8):909–15.

40. Sadjadieh G, Engstrøm T, Høfsten DE, et al. Bleeding events after ST-segment elevation myocardial infarction in patients randomized to an all-comer clinical trial compared with unselected patients. Am J Cardiol 2018;122(8):1287–96.

41. Buchtele N, Herkner H, Schörgenhofer C, et al. High platelet reactivity after transition from cangrelor to ticagrelor in hypothermic cardiac arrest survivors with ST-segment elevation myocardial infarction. J Clin Med 2020;9(2). https://doi.org/10.3390/jcm9020583.

42. Skorko A, Mumford A, Thomas M, et al. Platelet dysfunction after out of hospital cardiac arrest. Results from POHCAR: a prospective observational, cohort study. Resuscitation 2019;136:105–11.

43. Righetti S, Montemerlo E, Soffici F, et al. Outcomes related to antiplatelet therapy in a high-risk ST-segment elevation myocardial infarction population: a retrospective real-world analysis of an Italian ECMO center. J Cardiovasc Pharmacol Ther 2020; 25(3):219–25.

44. Bednar F, Kroupa J, Ondrakova M, et al. Antiplatelet efficacy of P2Y12 inhibitors (prasugrel, ticagrelor, clopidogrel) in patients treated with mild therapeutic hypothermia after cardiac arrest due to acute myocardial infarction. J Thromb Thrombolysis 2016;41(4):549–55.

45. Schüpke S, Neumann F-J, Menichelli M, et al. Ticagrelor or prasugrel in patients with acute coronary syndromes. N Engl J Med 2019;381(16):1524–34.

46. Umińska JM, Ratajczak J, Buszko K, et al. Impact of mild therapeutic hypothermia on bioavailability of ticagrelor in patients with acute myocardial infarction after out-of-hospital cardiac arrest. Cardiol J 2019. https://doi.org/10.5603/CJ.a2019.0024.

47. Ratcovich H, Sadjadieh G, Andersson HB, et al. The effect of TIcagrelor administered through a nasogastric tube to COMAtose patients undergoing acute percutaneous coronary intervention: the TICOMA study. EuroIntervention 2017;12(14):1782–8.

48. Bhatt DL, Stone GW, Mahaffey KW, et al. Effect of platelet inhibition with cangrelor during PCI on ischemic events. N Engl J Med 2013;368(14):1303–13.

49. Stone GW, Généreux P, Harrington RA, et al. Impact of lesion complexity on peri-procedural adverse events and the benefit of potent intravenous platelet adenosine diphosphate receptor inhibition after percutaneous coronary intervention: core laboratory analysis from 10 854 patients from the CHAMPI. Eur Heart J 2018;39(46):4112–21.

50. Ouweneel DM, Eriksen E, Sjauw KD, et al. Percutaneous mechanical circulatory support versus intra-aortic balloon pump in cardiogenic shock after acute myocardial infarction. J Am Coll Cardiol 2017;69(3):278–87.

51. Grothusen C, Friedrich C, Attmann T, et al. Coronary artery bypass surgery within 48 hours after cardiac arrest due to acute myocardial infarction. Eur J Cardio-thoracic Surg 2017;52(2):297–302.

52. Anderson HV, Shaw RE, Brindis RG, et al. A contemporary overview of percutaneous coronary interventions. The American College of Cardiology-National Cardiovascular Data Registry (ACC-NCDR). J Am Coll Cardiol 2002;39(7):1096–103.

53. Mehta RH, Harjai KJ, Grines L, et al. Sustained ventricular tachycardia or fibrillation in the cardiac catheterization laboratory among patients receiving primary percutaneous coronary intervention: incidence, predictors, and outcomes. J Am Coll Cardiol 2004;43(10):1765–72.

54. Brennan JM, Curtis JP, Dai D, et al. Enhanced mortality risk prediction with a focus on high-risk percutaneous coronary intervention: results from 1,208,137 procedures in the NCDR (National Cardiovascular Data Registry). JACC Cardiovasc Interv 2013;6(8):790–9.

55. Wagner H, Terkelsen CJ, Friberg H, et al. Cardiac arrest in the catheterisation laboratory: a 5-year experience of using mechanical chest compressions to facilitate PCI during prolonged resuscitation efforts. Resuscitation 2010;81(4):383–7.

56. Wagner H, Hardig BM, Rundgren M, et al. Mechanical chest compressions in the coronary catheterization laboratory to facilitate coronary intervention and survival in patients requiring prolonged resuscitation efforts. Scand J Trauma Resusc Emerg Med 2016;24:4.

57. Venturini JM, Retzer E, Estrada JR, et al. Mechanical chest compressions improve rate of return of spontaneous circulation and allow for initiation of percutaneous circulatory support during cardiac arrest in the cardiac catheterization laboratory. Resuscitation 2017;115:56–60.

58. Derwall M, Brücken A, Bleilevens C, et al. Doubling survival and improving clinical outcomes using a left ventricular assist device instead of chest compressions for resuscitation after prolonged cardiac arrest: a large animal study. Crit Care 2015;19(1):123.

59. Shawl FA, Domanski MJ, Wish MH, et al. Emergency cardiopulmonary bypass support in patients with cardiac arrest in the catheterization laboratory. Cathet Cardiovasc Diagn 1990;19(1):8–12.

60. Zanuttini D, Armellini I, Nucifora G, et al. Impact of emergency coronary angiography on in-hospital outcome of unconscious survivors after out-of-hospital cardiac arrest. Am J Cardiol 2012;110(12):1723–8.

61. Yannopoulos D, Bartos JA, Martin C, et al. Minnesota resuscitation consortium's advanced perfusion and reperfusion cardiac life support strategy for out-of-hospital refractory ventricular fibrillation. J Am Heart Assoc 2016;5(6). https://doi.org/10.1161/JAHA.116.003732.

62. Yannopoulos D. The interventional cardiologist as a resuscitator: a new era of machines in the cardiac catheterization laboratory. Hellenic J Cardiol 2017;58(6):401–2.

63. Bartos JA, Doonan AL, Yannopoulos D. Identifying candidates for advanced hemodynamic support after cardiac arrest. Circulation 2018;137(3):283–5.

64. Wilson M, Grossestreuer AV, Gaieski DF, et al. Incidence of coronary intervention in cardiac arrest survivors with non-shockable initial rhythms and no evidence of ST-elevation MI (STEMI). Resuscitation 2017;113:83–6.

65. Taglieri N, Saia F, Bacchi Reggiani ML, et al. Prognostic significance of shockable and non-shockable cardiac arrest in ST-segment elevation myocardial infarction patients undergoing primary angioplasty. Resuscitation 2018;123:8–14.

66. Fothergill RT, Watson LR, Virdi GK, et al. Survival of resuscitated cardiac arrest patients with ST-elevation myocardial infarction (STEMI) conveyed directly to a Heart Attack Centre by ambulance clinicians. Resuscitation 2014;85(1):96–8.

67. Bartos JA, Carlson K, Carlson C, et al. Surviving refractory out-of-hospital ventricular fibrillation cardiac arrest: critical care and extracorporeal membrane oxygenation management. Resuscitation 2018;132:47–55.

68. Kosmopoulos M, Roukoz H, Sebastian P, et al. Increased QT dispersion is linked to worse outcomes in patients hospitalized for out-of-hospital cardiac arrest. J Am Heart Assoc 2020;9(16):e016485.

69. Slapnik E, Rauber M, Noc M, et al. Abstract 20034: outcome of conscious survivors of out-of-hospital cardiac arrest. Circulation 2017;136(suppl_1):A20034.

70. Otani T, Sawano H, Natsukawa T, et al. Global Registry of Acute Coronary Events risk score predicts mortality and neurological outcome in out-of-hospital cardiac arrest. Am J Emerg Med 2017;35(5):685–91.

71. Foley LM, Clark RSB, Vazquez AL, et al. Enduring disturbances in regional cerebral blood flow and brain oxygenation at 24 h after asphyxial cardiac arrest in developing rats. Pediatr Res 2017;81(1–1):94–8.

72. Ladejobi A, Pasupula DK, Adhikari S, et al. Implantable defibrillator therapy in cardiac arrest survivors with a reversible cause. Circ Arrhythm Electrophysiol 2018;11(3):e005940.

73. Boyce LW, Reinders CC, Volker G, et al. Out-of-hospital cardiac arrest survivors with cognitive impairments have lower exercise capacity. Resuscitation 2017;115:90–5.

74. Kim C, Jung H, Choi HE, et al. Cardiac rehabilitation after acute myocardial infarction resuscitated from cardiac arrest. Ann Rehabil Med 2014;38(6): 799–804.

75. Lilja G, Nilsson G, Nielsen N, et al. Anxiety and depression among out-of-hospital cardiac arrest survivors. Resuscitation 2015;97:68–75.

76. Piegza M, Jaszke M, Ścisło P, et al. Symptoms of depression and anxiety after cardiac arrest. Psychiatr Pol 2015;49(3):465–76.

77. Fordyce CB, Chen AY, Wang TY, et al. Patterns of use of targeted temperature management for acute myocardial infarction patients following out-of-hospital cardiac arrest: insights from the National Cardiovascular Data Registry. Am Heart J 2018;206:131–3.

78. Laitio R, Hynninen M, Arola O, et al. Effect of inhaled xenon on cerebral white matter damage in comatose survivors of out-of-hospital cardiac arrest: a randomized clinical trial. JAMA 2016;315(11): 1120–8.

79. Chisholm GE, Grejs A, Thim T, et al. Safety of therapeutic hypothermia combined with primary percutaneous coronary intervention after out-of-hospital cardiac arrest. Eur Heart J Acute Cardiovasc Care 2015;4(1):60–3.

80. Jacob M, Hassager C, Bro-Jeppesen J, et al. The effect of targeted temperature management on coagulation parameters and bleeding events after out-of-hospital cardiac arrest of presumed cardiac cause. Resuscitation 2015;96:260–7.

81. Shah N, Chaudhary R, Mehta K, et al. Therapeutic hypothermia and stent thrombosis: a nationwide analysis. JACC Cardiovasc Interv 2016;9(17): 1801–11.

82. Wiberg S, Kjaergaard J, Kjærgaard B, et al. The biomarkers neuron-specific enolase and S100b measured the day following admission for severe accidental hypothermia have high predictive values for poor outcome. Resuscitation 2017;121: 49–53.

83. Lee YH, Oh YT, Ahn HC, et al. The prognostic value of the grey-to-white matter ratio in cardiac arrest patients treated with extracorporeal membrane oxygenation. Resuscitation 2016;99:50–5.

84. Keijzer HM, Hoedemaekers CWE, Meijer FJA, et al. Brain imaging in comatose survivors of cardiac arrest: pathophysiological correlates and prognostic properties. Resuscitation 2018;133:124–36.

85. Peckham ME, Anderson JS, Rassner UA, et al. Low b-value diffusion weighted imaging is promising in the diagnosis of brain death and hypoxic-ischemic injury secondary to cardiopulmonary arrest. Crit Care 2018;22(1):165.

86. Cueni-Villoz N, Devigili A, Delodder F, et al. Increased blood glucose variability during therapeutic hypothermia and outcome after cardiac arrest. Crit Care Med 2011;39(10):2225–31.

87. Couper K, Kimani PK, Gale CP, et al. Patient, health service factors and variation in mortality following resuscitated out-of-hospital cardiac arrest in acute coronary syndrome: analysis of the Myocardial Ischaemia National Audit Project. Resuscitation 2018;124:49–57. https://doi.org/10.1016/j.resuscitation.2018.01.011.

88. Kroupa J, Knot J, Ulman J, et al. Characteristics and survival determinants in patients after out-of-hospital cardiac arrest in the era of 24/7 coronary intervention facilities. Heart Lung Circ 2017;26(8): 799–807.

89. Baek JY, Choi BG, Rha S-W, et al. Comparison of two-year outcomes of acute myocardial infarction caused by coronary artery spasm versus that caused by coronary atherosclerosis. Am J Cardiol 2019;124(10):1493–500.

90. Velibey Y, Parsova EC, Ceylan US, et al. Outcomes of survivors of ST-segment elevation myocardial infarction complicated by out-of-hospital cardiac arrest: a single-center surveillance study. Turk Kardiyol Dern Ars 2019;47(1):10–20.

91. Kvakkestad KM, Sandvik L, Andersen GØ, et al. Long-term survival in patients with acute myocardial infarction and out-of-hospital cardiac arrest: a prospective cohort study. Resuscitation 2018;122: 41–7.

92. Dicker B, Todd VF, Tunnage B, et al. Direct transport to PCI-capable hospitals after out-of-hospital cardiac arrest in New Zealand: inequities and outcomes. Resuscitation 2019;142:111–6.

93. Taglieri N, Saia F, Lanzillotti V, et al. Impact of a territorial ST-segment elevation myocardial infarction network on prognosis of patients with out-of-hospital cardiac arrest. Acute Card Care 2011; 13(3):143–7.

94. Valle JA, Ho PM. Excluding the elephant in the room: cardiac arrest. J Am Heart Assoc 2019;8(1): e011381.

95. Wang Y, Wang M, Ni Y, et al. Can systemic thrombolysis improve prognosis of cardiac arrest patients during cardiopulmonary resuscitation? A systematic review and meta-analysis. J Emerg Med 2019; 57(4):478–87.

96. Lebiedz P, Meiners J, Samol A, et al. Electrocardiographic changes during therapeutic hypothermia. Resuscitation 2012;83(5):602–6.

Diagnosis and Management of Late-presentation ST-elevation Myocardial Infarction and Complications

Joe Aoun, MD, Neal S. Kleiman, MD,
Sachin S. Goel, MD*

KEYWORDS

- Myocardial infarction complications • Late presentation • STEMI
- Percutaneous coronary interventions • Thrombolysis • Fibrinolysis • Mechanical complications

KEY POINTS

- Late ST-elevation myocardial infarction presentation is associated with higher incidence of mechanical complications and worse outcomes.
- Reperfusion strategy for symptomatic latecomers is indicated.
- Reperfusion strategy for asymptomatic latecomers is controversial and stress testing can guide management.
- In contrast to the American College of Cardiology/American Heart Association guidelines, the 2018 European Society of Cardiology/European Association for Cardiothoracic Surgery guidelines suggest consideration of routine primary percutaneous coronary intervention in late presenters (12–48 hours).

 Video content accompanies this article at http://www.interventional.theclinics.com.

BACKGROUND

Ischemic heart disease is the most common cause of mortality worldwide. ST-elevation myocardial infarction (STEMI) constitutes approximately 29% of acute coronary syndrome cases in the United States and 47% in Europe.[1,2] In North America and Europe, most patients are treated with percutaneous coronary interventions (PCI), given the availability and ease of access to catheterization laboratories in the current era. Fibrinolysis is also used in non–PCI-capable facilities and in certain uncommon situations. Despite the clarity of the algorithm for the management of early STEMI presenters, the appropriate treatment of latecomers is not as evident, and is accompanied by more complications, more use of mechanical circulatory support (MCS), and worse outcomes. Early intervention has decreased the risk of mechanical complications of myocardial infarction (MI), which are currently almost exclusively encountered among latecomers. This article summarizes the available evidence on management and complications of latecomers.

DEFINITION AND DIAGNOSIS

Late presentation of MI is not well defined. Hypothetically, the term early refers to patients whose MI is still evolving and who will clearly benefit from restoration of myocardial perfusion with subsequent lower morbidity and mortality. In contrast, late presentation does not necessarily preclude reperfusion therapy, but the management should be decided on a case-by-case basis. In the classic canine study, myocardial

Department of Cardiovascular Medicine, Houston Methodist DeBakey Heart & Vascular Center, 6550 Fannin Street, Suite 1901, Houston, TX 77030, USA
* Corresponding author. 6550 Fannin Street, Suite 18.53, Houston, TX 77030.
E-mail address: ssgoel@houstonmethodist.org

Intervent Cardiol Clin 10 (2021) 369–380
https://doi.org/10.1016/j.iccl.2021.03.008
2211-7458/21/© 2021 Elsevier Inc. All rights reserved.

salvage after 6 hours of coronary occlusion and reperfusion was thought to be minimal or even absent.[3] This model was roughly confirmed by the time-to-treatment analyses of the Second International Study of Infarct Survival (ISIS-2) of fibrinolysis with streptokinase.[4] Nevertheless, thrombolysis has proved to be efficacious up to 12 hours after STEMI. However, if administered beyond that period, the risk of hemorrhagic stroke and myocardial rupture seem to counterbalance the reduced benefit achieved by reperfusion of largely infarction myocardium, which has led to a general consensus that late presenters are patients who present more than 12 hours after symptom onset.[5–7] The proportion of patients presenting late varies between 8.5% and 40%.[8,9] Factors associated with late presentation include female sex, African American ethnicity, diabetes mellitus, prior coronary revascularization, lower income and lower level of education, and the country of origin (30% of patients are late presenters in India, for example).[10,11] More recently, during the coronavirus disease 2019 (COVID-19) pandemic, it has been hypothesized that the fear of contagion has also led to later presentation to hospitals.[12]

The diagnosis of late-presenting MI is based on history (time of symptom onset). However, the reported time of symptom onset cannot necessarily be correlated with the precise time of coronary occlusion. The physical examination occasionally offer hints toward late MI complications: hypotension, muffled heart sounds, and increased jugular venous distention are in favor of a myocardial free wall rupture with tamponade, and a new systolic murmur can be heard in the setting of a secondary ischemic mitral regurgitation or a ventricular septal defect. Electrocardiographic findings can also be helpful in the diagnosis. Within the first few minutes of a transmural MI, the T waves become peaked and rapidly evolve into ST segment elevation (Pardee sign). In general, latecomers present with Q waves in addition to ST elevation, which can evolve into T-wave inversion with an isoelectric ST segment. Q waves can persist indefinitely. Rarely, ST elevation persists along with the Q waves, implying the possibility of left ventricular aneurysm formation. In addition, transthoracic echocardiography is helpful in the diagnosis of MI complications along with their hemodynamic consequences.

REPERFUSION MANAGEMENT AND STRATEGIES

Acute coronary occlusion (usually thrombosis at the site of a disrupted plaque) causes time-dependent irreversible myocardial damage.[3] This concept has prompted early revascularization therapy in STEMI. Pharmacologic therapy for late MI is identical to early MI, although the utility of certain medications remains uncertain when given late. In particular, as thrombi age and become organized, fibrinolytic drugs may be less effective. The indication for revascularization of the infarct-related artery (IRA) depends on the duration of the artery's occlusion. Early reperfusion therapy (within first 12 hours of symptoms) is associated with a reduction in infarct size, preservation of left ventricular function, and prolonged survival.[13,14] Reperfusion strategy for latecomers (between 12 hours and 3 months) remains controversial.

The open-artery hypothesis suggests that late mechanical revascularization of an IRA supplying a necrotic myocardium may limit infarct size and remodeling, reduce electrical instability, and also may provide supplemental blood supply to that area via collaterals and provide survival benefit.[15] The proposed hypothesis is the basis of multiple basic and clinical studies attempting to determine the benefit of revascularization in latecomers.

In a canine model (free of atherosclerosis), acute coronary occlusion leads to abrupt decrease in coronary blood flow, seen mainly in the subendocardial region compared with the subepicardial or the marginal ischemic areas.[16] Over time, the blood flow increases progressively to achieve 46% and 76% of baseline flow at 48 and 96 hours, respectively. The flow restoration is related to an improved supply by collateral vasculature.[16] These findings are not related to spontaneous revascularization, because the arteries remained mechanically occluded in experimental models. It has been suggested that coronary flow rate as low as 0.05 to 0.1 mL/min/g can maintain viability of the ischemic territory.[16] In addition, another study suggests that mitochondrial and cellular function, as well as cell integrity, can be maintained with only 20% of the baseline coronary blood flow (estimated at 0.2 mL/min/g of myocardial tissue).[17] The clinical course of an acute MI differs from experimentally provoked acute coronary occlusion. Subtotal occlusions, spontaneous resolution, and recanalization of coronary lesions are seen in as many as 34% of patients undergoing coronary angiography post-MI.[18] This phenomenon may be seen more often in latecomers, in up to 50% of the cases.[19–21] Spontaneous resolution is associated with improved outcomes compared with patients without reperfusion therapy.[22–24] In addition, recurrent occlusions in the same vessel may lead to preconditioning of myocardium, resulting in resistance to necrosis even with subsequent prolonged periods of ischemia.[25] Conceivably, these considerations may offer a framework to consider revascularization in latecomers as a result of preservation of the myocardium by collateral blood vessels, a preconditioning effect induced by cyclic flow variations and the existence of preconditioned myocardium. The extrapolation of these findings into clinically relevant outcomes such as reduction in deaths or recurrent MIs has been investigated in large clinical randomized controlled trials.

THROMBOLYSIS IN LATE ST-ELEVATION MYOCARDIAL INFARCTION

Early fibrinolytic therapy reduces mortality in STEMI (relative risk reduction of 51%, 26%, and 20% if administered within the first hour, 3 hours, or between 3 and 6 hours respectively compared with 6 and 12 hours).[26] The EMERAS (Estudio Multicentrico Estreptoquinasa Republicas de America del Sur) and the LATE (Late Assessment of Thrombolytic Efficacy) trials showed the efficacy of fibrinolytics when given within 12 hours of symptom onset but failed to prove any benefit in latecomers (between 12 and 24 hours).[5,6] In contrast, a subgroup of latecomers (in the LATE study) with ongoing symptoms and/or significant electrocardiographic changes still had a relative risk reduction of 22% in mortality. Furthermore, the ISIS-2 trial also showed a reduction in mortality by 19% in patients receiving streptokinase between 12 and 24 hours from symptom onset.[4]

- According to the 2013 American College of Cardiology Foundation (ACCF)/American Heart Association (AHA) guidelines, in a non–PCI-capable facility (>120 minutes from door to transfer to balloon), patients with early presentation (<12 hours) should be treated with fibrinolytics (class I, level of evidence [LOE] A). In latecomers (12–24 hours) with evidence of ongoing ischemia, hemodynamic instability, or those with large area of myocardium at risk, fibrinolytics are reasonable (class IIa, LOE C).[27] After administration of thrombolytics, patients should be transferred to a PCI-capable facility. There is no indication for thrombolysis in asymptomatic latecomers or patients with very late presentation beyond 24 hours from symptom onset.

PERCUTANEOUS CORONARY INTERVENTIONS IN LATE ST-ELEVATION MYOCARDIAL INFARCTION

Percutaneous coronary intervention has also been studied in latecomers. Coronary artery stenting with a drug-eluting stent is the recommended intervention. Routine thrombus aspiration in late presenters (12–48 hours) has failed to improve mortality or major adverse cardiac events.[28] The PL-ACS (Polish Registry of Acute Coronary Syndromes) study based on the Polish registry of acute coronary syndromes showed that 8.6% (2036 out of 23,517) of STEMI patients were latecomers (12–24 hours). Around 45% of these patients underwent coronary angiography, of whom 92% underwent reperfusion by PCI. The invasive approach was associated with a lower mortality at 12 months compared with conservative management (9.3% vs 17.9%, $P<.0001$).[9]

Several studies have addressed outcomes of different management strategies in both symptomatic and asymptomatic late presentations of MI. The outcomes of invasive reperfusion strategy in symptomatic latecomers (12–72 hours, N = 58) were compared with early presenters (<12 hours, N = 807) by Nepper-Christensen and colleagues.[29] At baseline, both groups had similar myocardial area at risk (34% ± 12% vs 33% ± 12%, $P = .37$) and were evaluated by cardiac magnetic resonance (CMR). At 3 months, CMR showed a larger infarct size (13% vs 11%; $P = .037$), lower left ventricular ejection fraction (52% vs 60%; $P<.001$), and a lower myocardial salvage index (0.58 vs 0.65; $P = .021$) in the latecomers group. Note that myocardial salvage of 50% or more was detected in around 65% of latecomers, indicating that late PCI may be beneficial in symptomatic patients.[29] Similar findings were noted using myocardial perfusion scan with a myocardial salvage index of 44% (23–73) in latecomers.[30]

Asymptomatic latecomers (12–48 hours, N = 365) were studied in the BRAVE-2 (Beyond 12 hours Reperfusion AlternatiVe Evaluation) trial, which randomized 182 patients to an invasive strategy (PCI with coronary stent with use of abciximab) and 183 patients to conservative medical management. The primary end point, left ventricular infarct size assessed using single-photon emission computed tomography (SPECT) imaging, was significantly smaller in the invasive group (8% vs 13%, $P<.001$)

compared with the conservative group. PCI-treated patients had no significant reduction in the composite of death, MI, and stroke at 30 days (4.4% vs 6.6%, P = .37).[19] A subsequent analysis of the trial at the 4-year follow-up, which included 88% of the patients, showed a significant mortality reduction of 45%.[31] A limitation of this study is the lack of power to assess mortality benefit with PCI in this population, in addition to the use of SPECT rather than cardiac MRI for assessment of infarct size.

The Occluded Artery Trial (OAT) enrolled 2166 stable patients presenting with late STEMI and a totally occluded IRA (between 3 and 28 days) and assigned them to either optimal medical therapy (OMT) alone or PCI with OMT.[32] Although the study population differs from the latecomers' population described earlier, it does help establish an upper period within which myocardial salvage can be obtained. Entry into this study excluded patients with ongoing ischemia at rest or cardiogenic shock. There was no difference in the composite outcome of all-cause mortality, nonfatal MI, or New York Heart Association (NYHA) class IV heart failure, 17.2% versus 15.6% (hazard ratio [HR], 1.16; 95% confidence interval [CI], 0.92–1.45; P = .20) or in each individual outcome. However, there was a trend toward excess reinfarction during 4 years of follow-up in the PCI group.[32] Total Occlusion Study of Canada 2 (TOSCA-2), an ancillary analysis of the OAT, showed that the PCI group maintained an IRA patency of 83% at 1 year without improvement in left ventricular systolic function.[33]

Silent ischemia after a recent MI was examined by in the SWISSI-II (Swiss Interventional Study on Silent Ischemia Type II) trial.[34] The study investigated 1057 patients who had a documented STEMI or non-STEMI within the preceding 3 months. Five-hundred and seventy-seven patients underwent bicycle exercise stress imaging, among whom 201 were eligible for randomization to either PCI or anti-ischemic drug therapy alone. Eligible patients had to be asymptomatic during the stress test but showed electrical and imaging signs of 1-vessel to 2-vessel ischemia and did not have triple-vessel disease on coronary angiograms. Major adverse cardiac events occurred less frequently in the PCI group (27 events) versus the OMT group (67 events) (HR, 0.33; 95% CI, 0.20–0.55; P<.001). Cardiac death was significantly improved with PCI (HR, 0.19; 95% CI, 0.05–0.67; P = .01) with a trend of benefit in all-cause mortality (HR, 0.42, 95% CI, 0.16–1.11; P = .08).[34] This population is slightly different than the latecomers population described previously. These patients have survived a previous nonrevascularized MI and still have residual provoked ischemia. Nevertheless, it highlights the benefit of revascularization in patients with residual ischemia.

In light of conflicting results regarding benefit of late reperfusion, Abbate, Appleton, and co-workers[35,36] performed a meta-analysis of randomized studies comparing late PCI (>12 hours after symptom onset) versus conservative medical management in hemodynamically stable patients. The final analysis included 10 randomized studies (including the OAT trial) and found that late PCI was associated with improved survival (OR, 0.49; 95% CI, 0.26–0.94; P = .03) and cardiac remodeling (an increase in left ventricular ejection fraction by 3.1%; 95% CI, 1.0–5.2; P = .0004). The greatest benefit was seen in symptomatic patients, those with residual ischemia and documented viability, and those with subtotal IRA occlusions.

- According to the 2013 ACCF/AHA guidelines, in a PCI-capable facility, all patients with a STEMI and ischemic symptoms of less than 12 hours from presentation should undergo PCI (class I, LOE A). Latecomers (12–24 hours) with evidence of ongoing ischemia (symptomatic) are to be considered for PCI (class IIa, LOE B). If the patient is in cardiogenic shock, PCI is recommended regardless of the time of symptoms onset (class I, LOE B)[27]. Delayed PCI (>24 hours) in asymptomatic stable patients with 1 or 2 diseased vessels and an occluded infarct artery without evidence of ischemia, should not be performed because of risk of harm (class III, LOE B).
- Similarly, the 2018 ESC/EACTS guidelines recommend PCI in late-presenting patients (>12 hours) with signs or symptoms of ischemia, hemodynamic instability, or life-threatening arrhythmias (class I, LOE C)[37]. In patients presenting days later, if symptoms are recurrent or silent ischemia is documented (on stress testing), revascularization may be considered. The main difference with the ACC/AHA is that the European guidelines suggest consideration of routine primary PCI in late presenters (12–48 hours) (class IIa, LOE B).[37] This recommendation is based on 2 studies showing that there might be some benefit in late revascularization (between

12–48 hours), even in asymptomatic patients.[19,30]

Using these guidelines, the authors suggest the algorithm for management of late STEMI presented in Fig. 1.

LATE-PRESENTATION MYOCARDIAL INFARCTION COMPLICATIONS: DIAGNOSIS AND MANAGEMENT

Cardiogenic Shock

Cardiogenic shock after MI (CS-MI) constitutes the most common cause of death post-MI. CS-MI is caused by left ventricular or right ventricular failure.

Left Ventricular Failure

Left ventricular failure post-MI is associated with a high risk of morbidity and mortality.[38] CS-MI occurs in about 80% of patients caused by pump failure when more than 40% of left ventricular mass is affected. CS-MI is associated with a 34.1% in-hospital mortality.[39] It can also result from mechanical complications of MI, such as ventricular septal defect, papillary muscle rupture, and free wall rupture.[38] CS-MI is more often encountered in the first 24 hours after the infarction, and it can therefore be the main presentation in latecomers with MI. Clinically, patients develop hypotension, shortness of breath, altered mental status, and/or end-organ damage. Physical examination findings can include an S3 gallop and bibasilar crackles. Latecomers with CS-MI and end-organ damage have worse outcomes. Management of CS-MI should be aimed at early reperfusion (preferably PCI) of the culprit vessel regardless of the timing of presentation, because it is associated with improved mortality.[40] As opposed to STEMI without cardiogenic shock, the intervention on the nonculprit lesion in CS-MI is not associated with lower rates of death from any cause or renal replacement therapy compared with culprit lesion–only PCI: 158 (45.9%) for culprit-alone group versus 189 (55.4%) for nonculprit group (relative risk, 0.83; 95% CI, 0.71–0.96; $P = .01$).[41] Pharmacological and mechanical support (left ventricular assist devices or intra-aortic balloon pumps) should be used when clinically indicated. Ongoing studies are evaluating the optimal timing and role of percutaneous left ventricular assist devices and extracorporeal membrane oxygenation.

Right Ventricular Failure

Right ventricle (RV) failure is mainly related to complete occlusion of the proximal right coronary artery and is seen in a third of patients with inferior STEMI. Isolated RV dysfunction is rare. RV-related CS-MI, similar to left ventricle (LV) failure, has a high mortality.[42] With ischemia, systolic RV dysfunction and reduced RV cardiac output lead to a decrement in the total cardiac output. Furthermore, ischemia causes right ventricular diastolic dysfunction, which increases right-sided filling pressure, further decreasing the filling of the RV and LV. Clinically, patients present with hypotension, increased jugular venous distention, and clear lung fields. Electrocardiographic findings include ST elevation in V1 and V4R, which are usually associated with an inferior STEMI (ST elevation in II, III, and AVF).[43] Echocardiography shows low RV ejection fraction, S' on tissue Doppler imaging, tricuspid annular plane systolic excursion, fractional area change, and the right ventricular index of myocardial performance. Because of the decreased contractility of the RV, the ventricle becomes preload and afterload dependent, so clinicians should be cautious with diuresis and tolerate higher central venous pressures.

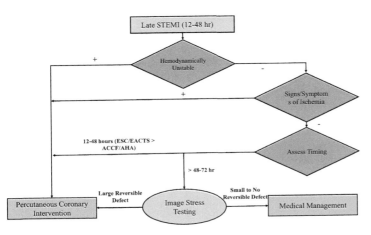

Fig. 1. Late STEMI management algorithm.

Nitrates, morphine, and β-blockers should be avoided. The management consists of early revascularization, inotropes, mechanical support (RV assist devices), and afterload reduction (pulmonary vasodilators) if needed.[44] Temporary pacemakers are used in the setting of atrioventricular block, but permanent pacemakers are less likely to be required.

Mechanical Complications of Myocardial Infraction

Although uncommon, mechanical complications of STEMI (MC-MI) increase significantly the in-hospital mortality to more than 40%.[45] In the current era, MC-MI occur in around 0.27% to 0.9% of patients with STEMI and are associated with higher rates of acute kidney injury, hemodialysis, longer length of stay, and use of MCS in up to 50% of patients.[45,46] Late presentation and late revascularization are associated with a higher incidence of MC-MI.[47] In case of MC-MI, female sex, increased age, obesity, and peripheral arterial disease are associated with higher rates of mortality.[45] The diagnosis is easier with advances in multimodality cardiac imaging techniques; however, a low threshold of suspicion is still required by physicians. Reperfusion therapy has been shown to reduce these complications, with invasive coronary interventions being superior to thrombolysis.[46,48–50] The use of MCS has not been shown to reduce mortality. Whether this is caused by MCS use in the sicker patients or related to their complications remains unclear. The APEX-AMI (Assessment of Pexelizumab in Acute Myocardial Infarction) study showed that surgical management increased survival from 33% to 68.8% at 90 days.[51]

Ventricular Septal Defect

Ventricular septal defect (VSD) is one of the most frequent MC-MI, with an estimated frequency of 1% to 3% of MIs, but the incidence has decreased to 0.17% to 0.26% with reperfusion therapy.[46,51,52] Typically, VSDs are diagnosed within the first 14 days post-MI and have a bimodal peak: within the first 24 hours and between day 3 and 5.[52] Clinically, the patient experiences worsening shortness of breath and hypotension. The physical examination is remarkable for a harsh systolic murmur inversely proportionate to the size of the defect, jugular venous distention, an S3 sound and other signs of left-sided heart failure. The diagnosis is based on clinical suspicion followed by confirmation with echocardiography (Video 1). Color flow Doppler identifies a left to right shunt through the ventricular septum and noninvasively quantifies the shunt (Qp/Qs, using the

left and right ventricular outflow tract time-velocity integrals). Although not required for diagnosis, a right heart catheterization shows a step-up in oxygen saturation at the RV level, increased c-v waves at the wedge position, and invasively quantifies the shunt (Qp/Qs, using Fick and Flamm formulas). The overall in-hospital mortality of patients with VSD is around 50%.[53] Predictors for worse outcomes include female sex, renal failure, diabetes, and elderly status.[45,54] A multidisciplinary heart team approach should be instituted in order to guide management. Pharmacologic therapy is used to stabilize patients until a surgical repair can be undertaken. Vasodilators (nitrates, nitroprusside) should be initiated unless contraindicated in order to reduce afterload and decrease the shunt flow. Inotropes can be used for support when required. A pulmonary arterial catheter can help guide these decisions. Severely ill patients can be treated with intra-aortic balloon pump placement as a bridge to surgery. Emergency surgical repair has been proved to decrease mortality in patients who underwent fibrinolysis or PCI, although it is crucial to note that critically sick patients might have been managed conservatively (Video 2).[45,54] Early surgical intervention is associated with a higher rate of VSD recurrence; the fresh necrotic tissue is very fragile and may not hold the sutures in position. In contrast, in stable patients, surgery is postponed for a few weeks until infarct site fibrosis occurs and necrosis becomes organized. Late closure of the VSD yields better surgical outcomes and improved long-term mechanical resistance of the tissue. Percutaneous closure device implantation is an alternative to surgery; nevertheless, clinical experience is more limited and residual shunts are common (complete closure 23%, partial closure 62%, failure to close 15%).[55]

Ventricular Free Wall Rupture

Ventricular free wall rupture occurs in less than 1% of MIs and constitutes the cause of 8% to 26% of deaths post-MI (Fig. 2). PCI has reduced the incidence of this complication, whereas fibrinolysis did not. Rupture occurs more often with left ventricular anterior and lateral wall infarcts. Other risk factors include older age, female sex, hypertension, first and single-vessel MI, absence of collaterals, and late administration of thrombolytics (>14 hours after presentation).[48,56–59] The time course is identical to VSDs with a bimodal peak. Clinically, patients develop pleuritic chest pain, increasing shortness of breath, hypotension, and sudden cardiac death. The physical examination is remarkable for muffled heart sounds, increased jugular

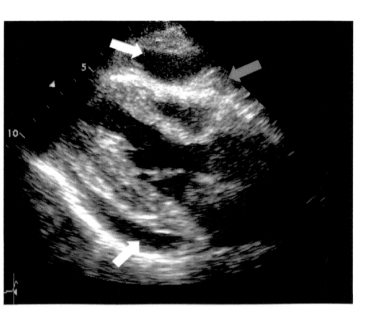

Fig. 2. Cardiac tamponade secondary to ventricular free wall rupture. White arrows indicate pericardial effusion; red arrows indicate blood coagulum.

venous distention, hypotension, pulsus paradoxus, electromechanical dissociation, and shock. The diagnosis is based on clinical suspicion, ST and T wave changes, and echocardiographic findings. Pericardial effusion is identified with increased acoustic echoes raising suspicion for blood coagulum and LV rupture site, in addition to tamponade features (early diastolic collapse of the RV, septal bounce, decreased mitral and tricuspid inflow, expiratory diastolic reversal of the hepatic veins). Right-heart catheterization shows equalization of diastolic pressures in cardiac chambers and a decreased y descent. Free-wall rupture can be lethal in around 60% to 90% of cases.[44,45] Cardiac surgical repair, with direct suture or placement of a patch, should be performed immediately.[60] In one-third of patients, a thrombus forms promptly in the pericardial space and seals the LV tear. Eventually, a small cavity forms (pseudoaneurysm) in the pericardial space, which communicates with the LV cavity via a narrow neck (Fig. 3). Pseudoaneurysms can rupture in half of untreated cases, making prompt surgical repair necessary.[61]

Rupture of a Papillary Muscle

Rupture of a papillary muscle occurs in around 1% of MIs. It can be partial or total.[62] The posteromedial muscle has a singular blood supply and is therefore more frequently affected than the anterolateral. The usual time course is bimodal, identical to other MC-MIs. Clinically,

patients report sudden onset of shortness of breath, as well as hypotension. The physical examination consists of a systolic murmur at the apex that can also radiate to the axillary line, along with signs of left-sided heart failure. Echocardiography shows a hyperdynamic LV with a flail papillary muscle, as opposed to ischemic mitral regurgitation related to regional wall motion abnormalities (Videos 3 and 4). Color flow Doppler may underestimate the degree of mitral regurgitation, which is mainly related to a rapid equalization in pressures between the LV and the left atrium. Pulmonary arterial catheterization shows a tall v wave and no oxygen step-up. Intra-aortic balloon pumps are sometimes used as a temporizing measure while awaiting definitive surgical repair.

Left Ventricular Aneurysm

Left ventricular aneurysm (true aneurysm) occurs in fewer than 5% of MIs and is associated most frequently with anterior and apical infarcts. The infarcted muscle progresses to a thin-walled dyskinetic area that expands with time secondary to intraventricular pressure. Timely reperfusion has decreased the incidence of this complication. Persistence of ST elevation is an indication of LV aneurysm formation. True aneurysms have a wide neck on echocardiography as opposed to a narrow neck seen with pseudoaneurysms. Patients with LV aneurysm have a higher mortality, which is thought to be related to ventricular arrhythmias.[63] Moreover, stasis

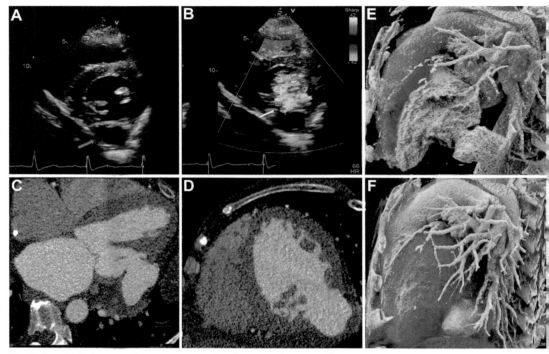

Fig. 3. Basal inferior pseudoaneurysm visualized on transthoracic echocardiogram (A, B), two-dimensional electro-cardiogram (ECG)-gated computed tomography (CT) (C, D) and three-dimensional volume rendering ECG-gated CT (E, F). Red arrow indicates pseudoaneurysm; white arrow indicates Doppler flow into the pseudoaneurysm. (Credits to Dr. Su Min Chang at DeBakey Heart & Vascular Center.)

along with endocardial inflammation creates a niche for intraventricular thrombosis formation. With the use of antithrombotic regimens, the incidence of LV thrombus has decreased. In most patients, LV thrombus is found incidentally on echocardiography (Fig. 4, Video 5). The use of contrast image enhancers can better detect the mural thrombus and facilitate the diagnosis. Cardiac MRI has a better sensitivity and helps predict the risk for embolism. Patients are at higher risk of systemic embolization (in up to 10%) and anticoagulation for 3 to 6 months is crucial.[64] Vitamin K antagonists are the mainstay of therapy; nevertheless, multiple successful

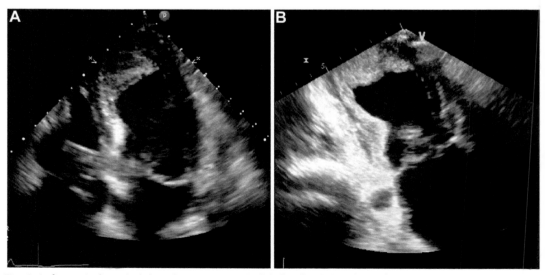

Fig. 4. Left ventricular apical thrombus seen on apical 4-chamber (A) and apical 2-chamber (B) views.

off-label uses of direct oral anticoagulants have been documented.[65]

OTHER COMPLICATIONS

Pericardial Complications

Pericardial complications of MI can range from pericarditis and pericardial effusion (hemopericardium, described earlier) to Dressler syndrome. Pericarditis can occur as early as the first day after the MI and as late as 8 weeks, but its incidence is decreasing with reperfusion therapies.[66] A pericardial friction rub can be heard. High-dose aspirin remains the treatment of choice because nonsteroidal antiinflammatory drugs and corticosteroids should be avoided.[67] Dressler syndrome, post–cardiac injury syndrome, or postpericardiotomy syndrome occurs between 1 and 8 weeks and is thought to be related to an immunologic response. Patients develop fever, pericarditis-type chest pain, pericardial effusion, and increased white blood cell count. Treatment is similar to acute pericarditis.

Other post-MI complications include arrhythmias, venous thrombosis, pulmonary embolism, and reinfarction.

SUMMARY

Late presentation of STEMI is an important and common entity. Patients are at higher risk of developing life-threatening post-MI complications along with increased morbidity and mortality. Late presenters (12–24 hours from symptom onset) benefit from revascularization, but those with very late presentations (>72 hours) might require ischemia-driven revascularization. Future perspectives should address the prevention and therapeutic management of latecomers in order to decrease the rate of complications in this important subset of patients.

CLINICS CARE POINTS

- Latecomers after STEMI (12-24 hours) with evidence of ongoing ischemia (symptomatic) should be considered for PCI.

- Delayed PCI (>24 hours) in asymptomatic stable patients with 1 or 2 diseased vessels and an occluded infarct related artery without evidence of ischemia should not be performed due to risk of harm.

- In latecomers after STEMI who are asymptomatic, stress testing can help guide decisions regarding invasive management. Further data are required in this subset of patients.

- It is important to have a high index of suspicion for mechanical complications in latecomers after STEMI as these are associated with high morbidity and mortality.

DISCLOSURE

The authors have nothing to disclose.

SUPPLEMENTARY DATA

Supplementary data to this article can be found online at https://doi.org/10.1016/j.iccl.2021.03.008.

REFERENCES

1. Lloyd-Jones D, Adams R, Carnethon M, et al. Heart disease and stroke statistics–2009 update: a report from the American Heart Association Statistics Committee and Stroke Statistics Subcommittee. Circulation 2009;119:480–6.

2. Mandelzweig L, Battler A, Boyko V, et al. The second Euro Heart Survey on acute coronary syndromes: characteristics, treatment, and outcome of patients with ACS in Europe and the Mediterranean Basin in 2004. Eur Heart J 2006;27:2285–93.

3. Reimer KA, Lowe JE, Rasmussen MM, et al. The wavefront phenomenon of ischemic cell death. 1. Myocardial infarct size vs duration of coronary occlusion in dogs. Circulation 1977;56:786–94.

4. Randomised trial of intravenous streptokinase, oral aspirin, both, or neither among 17,187 cases of suspected acute myocardial infarction: ISIS-2. ISIS-2 (Second International Study of Infarct Survival) Collaborative Group. Lancet 1988;2:349–60.

5. Randomised trial of late thrombolysis in patients with suspected acute myocardial infarction. EMERAS (Estudio Multicéntrico Estreptoquinasa Repúblicas de América del Sur) Collaborative Group. Lancet 1993;342:767–72.

6. Late Assessment of Thrombolytic Efficacy (LATE) study with alteplase 6-24 hours after onset of acute myocardial infarction. Lancet 1993;342:759–66.

7. Becker RC, Charlesworth A, Wilcox RG, et al. Cardiac rupture associated with thrombolytic therapy: impact of time to treatment in the Late Assessment of Thrombolytic Efficacy (LATE) study. J Am Coll Cardiol 1995;25:1063–8.

8. Albrahim M, Ahmed AM, Alwakeel A, et al. Predictors of delayed pre-hospital presentation among patients with ST-segment elevation myocardial infarction. Qatar Med J 2016;2016:7.

9. Gierlotka M, Gasior M, Wilczek K, et al. Reperfusion by primary percutaneous coronary intervention in patients with ST-segment elevation myocardial infarction within 12 to 24 hours of the onset of symptoms (from a prospective national observational study [PL-ACS]). Am J Cardiol 2011;107: 501–8.

10. Rodrigues JA, Melleu K, Schmidt MM, et al. Independent predictors of late presentation in patients with ST-segment elevation myocardial infarction. Arq Bras Cardiol 2018;111:587–93.

11. McNair PW, Bilchick KC, Keeley EC. Very late presentation in ST elevation myocardial infarction: predictors and long-term mortality. Int J Cardiol Heart Vasc 2019;22:156–9.

12. Delayed STEMI Presentation During the COVID-19 Pandemic [Internet]. American College of Cardiology. Available at: https://www.acc.org/latest-in-cardiology/articles/2020/06/05/09/51/delayed-stemi-presentation-during-the-covid-19-pandemic. Accessed August 23, 2020.

13. Lavie CJ, O'Keefe JH, Chesebro JH, et al. Prevention of late ventricular dilatation after acute myocardial infarction by successful thrombolytic reperfusion. Am J Cardiol 1990;66:31–6.

14. Cohen M, Maritz F, Gensini GF, et al. The TETAMI trial: the safety and efficacy of subcutaneous enoxaparin versus intravenous unfractionated heparin and of tirofiban versus placebo in the treatment of acute myocardial infarction for patients not thrombolyzed: methods and design. J Thromb Thrombolysis 2000;10:241–6.

15. Braunwald E. Myocardial reperfusion, limitation of infarct size, reduction of left ventricular dysfunction, and improved survival. Should the paradigm be expanded? Circulation 1989;79:441–4.

16. Bishop SP, White FC, Bloor CM. Regional myocardial blood flow during acute myocardial infarction in the conscious dog. Circ Res 1976;38:429–38.

17. Anselmi M, Bolognese L, Chierchia S, et al. The role of myocardial viability in deriving benefit from reestablishing infarct-related artery flow after acute myocardial infarction. Prog Cardiovasc Dis 2000;42:455–70.

18. Schömig A, Kastrati A, Dirschinger J, et al. Coronary stenting plus platelet glycoprotein IIb/IIIa blockade compared with tissue plasminogen activator in acute myocardial infarction. Stent versus Thrombolysis for Occluded Coronary Arteries in Patients with Acute Myocardial Infarction Study Investigators. N Engl J Med 2000;343:385–91.

19. Schömig A, Mehilli J, Antoniucci D, et al. Mechanical reperfusion in patients with acute myocardial infarction presenting more than 12 hours from

symptom onset: a randomized controlled trial. JAMA 2005;293:2865–72.

20. DeWood MA, Spores J, Notske R, et al. Prevalence of total coronary occlusion during the early hours of transmural myocardial infarction. N Engl J Med 1980;303:897–902.

21. DeWood MA, Stifter WF, Simpson CS, et al. Coronary arteriographic findings soon after non-Q-wave myocardial infarction. N Engl J Med 1986;315:417–23.

22. Fefer P, Hod H, Hammerman H, et al. Relation of clinically defined spontaneous reperfusion to outcome in ST-elevation myocardial infarction. Am J Cardiol 2009;103:149–53.

23. Bainey KR, Fu Y, Granger CB, et al. Benefit of angiographic spontaneous reperfusion in STEMI: does it extend to diabetic patients? Heart 2009; 95:1331–6.

24. Bainey KR, Fu Y, Wagner GS, et al. Spontaneous reperfusion in ST-elevation myocardial infarction: comparison of angiographic and electrocardiographic assessments. Am Heart J 2008;156:248–55.

25. Kloner RA, Shook T, Antman EM, et al. Prospective temporal analysis of the onset of preinfarction angina versus outcome: an ancillary study in TIMI-9B. Circulation 1998;97:1042–5.

26. Effectiveness of intravenous thrombolytic treatment in acute myocardial infarction. Gruppo Italiano per lo Studio della Streptochinasi nell'Infarto Miocardico (GISSI). Lancet 1986;1:397–402.

27. O'Gara PT, Kushner FG, Ascheim DD, et al. 2013 ACCF/AHA guideline for the management of ST-elevation myocardial infarction: a report of the American College of Cardiology Foundation/ American Heart Association Task Force on Practice Guidelines. Circulation 2013;127:e362–425.

28. Freund A, Schock S, Stiermaier T, et al. Thrombus aspiration in patients with ST-elevation myocardial infarction presenting late after symptom onset: long-term clinical outcome of a randomized trial. Clin Res Cardiol 2019;108:1208–14.

29. Nepper-Christensen L, Lønborg J, Høfsten DE, et al. Benefit from reperfusion with primary percutaneous coronary intervention beyond 12 hours of symptom duration in patients with ST-segment-elevation myocardial infarction. Circ Cardiovasc Interv 2018;11:e006842.

30. Busk M, Kaltoft A, Nielsen SS, et al. Infarct size and myocardial salvage after primary angioplasty in patients presenting with symptoms for <12 h vs. 12-72 h. Eur Heart J 2009;30:1322–30.

31. Ndrepepa G, Kastrati A, Mehilli J, et al. Mechanical reperfusion and long-term mortality in patients with acute myocardial infarction presenting 12 to 48 hours from onset of symptoms. JAMA 2009;301: 487–8.

32. Hochman JS, Lamas GA, Buller CE, et al. Coronary intervention for persistent occlusion after

myocardial infarction. N Engl J Med 2006;355: 2395–407.

33. Dzavík V, Buller CE, Lamas GA, et al. Randomized trial of percutaneous coronary intervention for subacute infarct-related coronary artery occlusion to achieve long-term patency and improve ventricular function: the Total Occlusion Study of Canada (TOSCA)-2 trial. Circulation 2006;114:2449–57.

34. Erne P, Schoenenberger AW, Burckhardt D, et al. Effects of percutaneous coronary interventions in silent ischemia after myocardial infarction: the SWISSI II randomized controlled trial. JAMA 2007; 297:1985–91.

35. Appleton DL, Abbate A, Biondi-Zoccai GGL. Late percutaneous coronary intervention for the totally occluded infarct-related artery: a meta-analysis of the effects on cardiac function and remodeling. Catheter Cardiovasc Interv 2008;71: 772–81.

36. Abbate A, Biondi-Zoccai GGL, Appleton DL, et al. Survival and cardiac remodeling benefits in patients undergoing late percutaneous coronary intervention of the infarct-related artery: evidence from a meta-analysis of randomized controlled trials. J Am Coll Cardiol 2008;51:956–64.

37. Neumann F-J, Sousa-Uva M, Ahlsson A, et al. 2018 ESC/EACTS guidelines on myocardial revascularization. Eur Heart J 2019;40:87–165.

38. Thiele H, Ohman EM, Desch S, et al. Management of cardiogenic shock. Eur Heart J 2015;36:1223–30.

39. Venkatason P, Zubairi YZ, Wan Ahmad WA, et al. In-hospital mortality of cardiogenic shock complicating ST-elevation myocardial infarction in Malaysia: a retrospective analysis of the Malaysian National Cardiovascular Database (NCVD) registry. BMJ Open 2019;9. Available at: https://www.ncbi. nlm.nih.gov/pmc/articles/PMC6502239/. Accessed November 2, 2020.

40. Hochman JS, Sleeper LA, Webb JG, et al. Early revascularization in acute myocardial infarction complicated by cardiogenic shock. SHOCK Investigators. Should we emergently revascularize occluded coronaries for cardiogenic shock. N Engl J Med 1999;341:625–34.

41. Thiele H, Akin I, Sandri M, et al. PCI strategies in patients with acute myocardial infarction and cardiogenic shock. N Engl J Med 2017;377: 2419–32.

42. Goldstein JA. Acute right ventricular infarction. Cardiol Clin 2012;30:219–32.

43. Wellens HJ. The value of the right precordial leads of the electrocardiogram. N Engl J Med 1999;340: 381–3.

44. Kinch JW, Ryan TJ. Right ventricular infarction. N Engl J Med 1994;330:1211–7.

45. Elbadawi A, Elgendy IY, Mahmoud K, et al. Temporal trends and outcomes of mechanical complications in patients with acute myocardial infarction. JACC Cardiovasc Interv 2019;12: 1825–36.

46. López-Sendón J, Gurfinkel EP, Lopez de Sa E, et al. Factors related to heart rupture in acute coronary syndromes in the global registry of acute coronary events. Eur Heart J 2010;31:1449–56.

47. Figueras J, Cortadellas J, Calvo F, et al. Relevance of delayed hospital admission on development of cardiac rupture during acute myocardial infarction: study in 225 patients with free wall, septal or papillary muscle rupture. J Am Coll Cardiol 1998;32: 135–9.

48. Bates ER. Reperfusion therapy reduces the risk of myocardial rupture complicating ST-elevation myocardial infarction. J Am Heart Assoc 2014;3: e001368.

49. Figueras J, Alcalde O, Barrabés JA, et al. Changes in hospital mortality rates in 425 patients with acute ST-elevation myocardial infarction and cardiac rupture over a 30-year period. Circulation 2008; 118:2783–9.

50. Moreno R, López-Sendón J, García E, et al. Primary angioplasty reduces the risk of left ventricular free wall rupture compared with thrombolysis in patients with acute myocardial infarction. J Am Coll Cardiol 2002;39:598–603.

51. French JK, Hellkamp AS, Armstrong PW, et al. Mechanical complications after percutaneous coronary intervention in ST-elevation myocardial infarction (from APEX-AMI). Am J Cardiol 2010;105:59–63.

52. Antman EM, Anbe DT, Armstrong PW, et al. ACC/AHA guidelines for the management of patients with ST-elevation myocardial infarction—executive summary. a report of the American College of Cardiology/American Heart Association Task Force on Practice Guidelines (Writing Committee to revise the 1999 guidelines for the management of patients with acute myocardial infarction). J Am Coll Cardiol 2004;44:671–719.

53. Moreyra AE, Huang MS, Wilson AC, et al. Trends in incidence and mortality rates of ventricular septal rupture during acute myocardial infarction. Am J Cardiol 2010;106:1095–100.

54. Crenshaw BS, Granger CB, Birnbaum Y, et al. Risk factors, angiographic patterns, and outcomes in patients with ventricular septal defect complicating acute myocardial infarction. GUSTO-I (Global Utilization of Streptokinase and TPA for Occluded Coronary Arteries) Trial Investigators. Circulation 2000; 101:27–32.

55. Calvert PA, Cockburn J, Wynne D, et al. Percutaneous closure of postinfarction ventricular septal defect: in-hospital outcomes and long-term

follow-up of UK experience. Circulation 2014;129: 2395–402.

56. Becker RC, Gore JM, Lambrew C, et al. A composite view of cardiac rupture in the United States National Registry of Myocardial Infarction. J Am Coll Cardiol 1996;27:1321–6.

57. Honan MB, Harrell FE, Reimer KA, et al. Cardiac rupture, mortality and the timing of thrombolytic therapy: a meta-analysis. J Am Coll Cardiol 1990;16:359–67.

58. Slater J, Brown RJ, Antonelli TA, et al. Cardiogenic shock due to cardiac free-wall rupture or tamponade after acute myocardial infarction: a report from the SHOCK Trial Registry. Should we emergently revascularize occluded coronaries for cardiogenic shock? J Am Coll Cardiol 2000;36:1117–22.

59. McMullan MH, Maples MD, Kilgore TL, et al. Surgical experience with left ventricular free wall rupture. Ann Thorac Surg 2001;71:1894–8 [discussion: 1898–9].

60. Núñez L, de la Llana R, López Sendón J, et al. Diagnosis and treatment of subacute free wall ventricular rupture after infarction. Ann Thorac Surg 1983; 35:525–9.

61. Arsanjani R, Lohrmann G, Allen S, et al. A multi-modality approach to left ventricular aneurysms: true vs false. Am J Med 2016;129:e113–6.

62. Nishimura RA, Otto CM, Bonow RO, et al. 2014 AHA/ ACC guideline for the management of patients with valvular heart disease: executive summary: a report of the American College of Cardiology/American Heart Association Task Force on Practice Guidelines. J Am Coll Cardiol 2014;63:2438–88.

63. Wissner E, Stevenson WG, Kuck K-H. Catheter ablation of ventricular tachycardia in ischaemic and non-ischaemic cardiomyopathy: where are we today? A clinical review. Eur Heart J 2012;33: 1440–50.

64. Delewi R, Zijlstra F, Piek JJ. Left ventricular thrombus formation after acute myocardial infarction. Heart 2012;98:1743–9.

65. Fleddermann AM, Hayes CH, Magalski A, et al. Efficacy of direct acting oral anticoagulants in treatment of left ventricular thrombus. Am J Cardiol 2019;124:367–72.

66. Shahar A, Hod H, Barabash GM, et al. Disappearance of a syndrome: Dressler's syndrome in the era of thrombolysis. Cardiology 1994;85: 255–8.

67. Imazio M, Spodick DH, Brucato A, et al. Controversial issues in the management of pericardial diseases. Circulation 2010;121:916–28.

Fibrinolytic Therapy in Patients with Acute ST-elevation Myocardial Infarction

Chayakrit Krittanawong, MD[a], Joshua Hahn, MD[a],
Waleed Kayani, MD[a], Hani Jneid, MD, FSCAI[a,b],*

KEYWORDS

- Fibrinolytic • ST-segment myocardial infarction • Percutaneous coronary intervention • Heart

---

KEY POINTS

- Criteria for successful fibrinolysis includes resolution of chest discomfort or ischemic symptoms and resolution of ST segments by 70%.
- The timing of fibrinolytic therapy delivery is critical being administered within 30 minutes of first medical contact and within 10 minutes of STEMI confirmation.
- PCI after fibrinolysis is an important managment approach to consider and can be summariazed into three broad categories: pharmacoinvasive, facilitated PCI and rescue PCI.
- There are important limitations and contraindications to fibrinolytic therapies as well as complications which clinicians should be well-versed in prior to initiation.

In patients who present with ST-segment myocardial infarction (STEMI), fibrinolytic therapy serves as a therapeutic option when primary percutaneous coronary intervention (PCI) cannot be performed in a timely manner. Fibrinolytic therapy can reestablish coronary artery blood flow, leading to myocardial salvage, mortality benefit, and improved cardiovascular outcomes. The effectiveness of fibrinolytic therapy is time sensitive, and best outcomes are noted within the initial 2 hours after symptom onset, with the benefits diminishing markedly after 3 hours. The later a patient presents after symptom onset with STEMI (particularly after 3 hours), the higher consideration should be given to primary PCI, because the risks of fibrinolytic therapy may outweigh its benefits. A pharmacoinvasive strategy may be selectively used after acute STEMI, including at times of scarce health care resources as seen during the coronavirus disease 2019 (COVID-19) pandemic. Four fibrinolytic agents have been developed for clinical use in patients with STEMI. This article reviews the available medical literature regarding fibrinolytic therapy in STEMI and discusses practical considerations for clinicians.

PATHOPHYSIOLOGIC INSIGHTS AND MECHANISMS OF ACTION

A basic understanding of the pathophysiology of STEMI and the pharmacology of fibrinolytic therapy is important to appreciate its therapeutic effect. Complete thrombotic occlusion of a coronary artery leading to transmural ischemia is often precipitated by the disruption (eg, rupture, erosion) of a preexisting at-risk or vulnerable coronary atherosclerotic plaque.[1] This disruption leads to rapid platelet activation

---

Conflicts of interest: none.
Funding/support: There was no funding for this work.
Special populations: cardiogenic shock; COVID 19.
[a] Section of Cardiology, Baylor College of Medicine, 7200 Cambridge Street, Houston, TX 77030, USA;
[b] Interventional Cardiology Fellowship Program, Interventional Cardiology Research, Baylor College of Medicine, Interventional Cardiology, The Michael E. DeBakey VA Medical Center, MEDVAMC - 2002 Holcombe Boulevard, Cardiology 3C-320C, Houston, TX 77030, USA
* Corresponding author. MEDVAMC - 2002 Holcombe Boulevard, Cardiology 3C-320C, Houston, TX 77030.
E-mail address: jneid@bcm.edu

Intervent Cardiol Clin 10 (2021) 381–390
https://doi.org/10.1016/j.iccl.2021.03.011
2211-7458/21/© 2021 Elsevier Inc. All rights reserved.

and aggregation with the coagulation cascade, which produces complete vessel thrombosis.[2]

The human hemostatic and fibrinolytic systems continually interact in order to maintain vessel patency and respond to injury. Within the fibrinolytic system, plasminogen serves as a precursor to the active enzyme plasmin, which degrades fibrin (clots). Naturally occurring tissue plasminogen activator (t-PA) cleaves plasminogen to create active plasmin and regulates fibrin degradation.[3] Plasminogen is found on the surface of fibrin and freely in the blood stream. Newer fibrinolytics more selectively target fibrin-bound plasminogen to reduce unintended off-target effects. In a nutshell, fibrinolytic agents essentially augment natural clot degradation where thrombosis has occurred.

CLINICAL CONSIDERATIONS
Criteria for Successful Fibrinolysis
The following criteria are used to assess for successful fibrinolysis:

1. Resolution of chest discomfort or ischemic symptoms
2. Resolution of ST segments by 70%

Evidence of successful clinical reperfusion is important when assessing the response to fibrinolytics. Chest discomfort should be frequently reassessed because sudden resolution of chest discomfort may indicate recanalization of the coronary artery with a sensitivity and specificity of 34% and 83% respectively.[4,5] In addition, resolution of ST-segment elevation is an important indication of successful reperfusion. In the GISSI-2 (Gruppo Italiano per lo Studio della Sopravvivenza nell'Infarto miocardico acuto-2) trial, individuals with 50% or more of a decrease in the ST-segment elevation had improved short-term outcomes.[6] This finding was more pronounced in those with greater than 80% reduction in the ST segment. Some clinicians have reported that, in serial electrocardiograms (ECGs), the sum of ST-segment reduction of 20% to 50% corresponds to reperfusion with a reported sensitivity of 73% to 88% and specificity of 63% to 80%.[5]

Timing
The timing of fibrinolytic therapy delivery is critical; it should be administered within 30 minutes of first medical contact and within 10 minutes of STEMI confirmation.[7,8] A timely door-to-needle time (≤30 min) is an important performance measure for health care providers and systems.[9] Several studies have indicated that the administration of fibrinolytic therapy should be within the first 3 to 4 hours after onset of symptoms,[10–13] with the greatest survival benefit within the first 120 minutes.[12,14] Boersma and colleagues[12] observed mortality reduction in individuals who received fibrinolytic therapy within 2 hours compared with their counterparts treated after this time frame (44% [95% confidence interval (CI), 32, 53] vs 20% [15, 25]; $P = .001$).[12] Goldberg and colleagues[14] also found reduced risk of death during hospitalization, which decreased with time to therapy. Individuals who received therapy within 3 hours had the lowest adjusted odds ratio (OR) of death. Overall, evidence suggests that fibrinolytic therapy delivered 12 hours after symptom onset is not likely to have a mortality benefit.

Prehospital Fibrinolytic Therapy
The practice of prehospital fibrinolytic therapy administered by emergency medical services (EMS) for STEMI has been studied.[12,15–17] Welsh and colleagues[18] showed that time to treatment was significantly reduced in patients who received prehospital fibrinolytic therapy. Furthermore, in a large meta-analysis by Morrison and colleagues,[17] which included 6 randomized trials (n = 6434), prehospital fibrinolytic therapy reduced early mortality by 17% compared with in-hospital fibrinolytic therapy. This benefit is especially evident when administered in the first 2 hours of symptom onset. Hospital systems need to appropriately train EMS in ECG interpretation, ensure seamless ECG transmission capability, develop reperfusion checklists, ensure capability to deliver all STEMI recommended medications with a clear facility destination before implementing prehospital fibrinolytics.[12,17,19]

Percutaneous Coronary Intervention after Fibrinolytic Therapy
There are various uses of PCI after fibrinolytic therapy (Table 1). Patients who present to facilities not capable of PCI are often immediately transferred for primary PCI at another hospital; however, national data indicate that such patients only receive PCI within 120 minutes approximately 50% of the time.[20] Thus, various PCI strategies after fibrinolysis can be used to reduce total ischemic time and improve outcomes.

Pharmacoinvasive approach
The pharmacoinvasive approach to STEMI involves administering fibrinolytic with immediate

Table 1
Percutaneous coronary intervention strategies following fibrinolytic therapy

Therapeutic Strategy	Description	Clinical Indications	Time Frame	Comments
Pharmaco-invasive	Coronary angiography ± PCI following completed fibrinolytic therapy after immediate transfer from non–PCI-capable facility	• Treated with fibrinolysis therapy without complications • Clinical noninvasive evidence of successful reperfusion without hemodynamic instability or shock	3–24 h of fibrinolytic therapy	• Good evidence to support improved outcomes • Proceed with emergent PCI in the event of signs of reinfarction, fibrinolytic failure, sudden hemodynamic instability and so forth
Facilitated PCI	Planned immediate PCI following fibrinolytic therapy	Consider in high-risk individuals who have received fibrinolytic therapy without immediately available PCI and who have very low bleeding risk	≤120 min from fibrinolytic therapy	• High bleeding risk, especially in individuals >75 y old • Limited evidence to support routine practice • Can consider in very-high-risk individuals
Rescue PCI	PCI that is conducted after failed fibrinolytic therapy and persistent evidence of myocardial infarction	Consider in patients with persistent ischemic symptoms, shock, acute heart failure, pulmonary edema, or hemodynamic instability	≤12 h from failed fibrinolysis	• High mortality if unsuccessful • Good evidence to support intervention given mortality/CHF reduction compared with routine care

Abbreviation: CHF, congestive heart failure.

transfer to a PCI-capable facility and early routine PCI after fibrinolysis within 3 to 24 hours is performed. This approach is currently recommended by major guidelines and has become a preferred strategy in many non–PCI-capable medical centers.[7,8,21] The timing of PCI after fibrinolysis remains an area of debate, because wait times vary significantly between trials. However, most recommend waiting 3 hours from fibrinolysis before PCI and no longer than 24 hours. In the TRANSFER-AMI (The Trial of Routine Angioplasty and Stenting after Fibrinolysis to Enhance Reperfusion in Acute Myocardial Infarction) trial, there was significant improvement in the composite end point of incidence of death, reinfarction, recurrent ischemia,

new or worsening heart failure, or cardiogenic shock at 30 days in patients who received early PCI (within 6 hours) after fibrinolysis.[22] One meta-analysis showed a reduced combined end point of reinfarction or death at 6 to 12 months in individuals receiving pharmacoinvasive strategy.[23] Ultimately, the pharmacoinvasive approach is the standard recommendation and early PCI should be performed following successful fibrinolytic therapy within 3 to 24 hours.

Facilitated percutaneous coronary intervention

The term facilitated PCI describes an approach to STEMI that refers to administering fibrinolytics with planned immediate PCI within 2 to

3 hours. Some advantages of this approach are shorter time to reperfusion and total ischemic time. However, PCI within this 2-hour to 3-hour time frame has not always been shown to reduce infarct size or improve outcomes, and is associated with increased bleeding risk.[24–26] The ASSENT-4 PCI (Assessment of the Safety and Efficacy of a New Treatment Strategy with Percutaneous Coronary Intervention) trial showed that facilitated PCI resulted in higher rates of the composite end point of death or heart failure or shock at 30 days compared with primary PCI.[24] Of note, secondary analysis has suggested that certain high-risk individuals presenting to non–PCI-capable centers may benefit more from a facilitated PCI approach.[26] Ultimately, the pharmacoinvasive approach of waiting 3 hours after fibrinolytic therapy for PCI is generally preferred; however, facilitated PCI within 2 to 3 hours from fibrinolytic therapy can be considered in very-high-risk individuals.

Rescue percutaneous coronary intervention

For patients who have failed fibrinolytic therapy for STEMI, rescue PCI should be pursued. By definition, rescue PCI is performed within 12 hours of failed fibrinolysis. Evidence of failed fibrinolysis includes persistent chest pain, worsening ST-segment elevation, heart failure, and/or hemodynamic instability. In the RESCUE (Randomized Comparison of Rescue Angioplasty With Conservative Management of Patients With Early Failure of Thrombolysis for Acute Anterior Myocardial Infarction) trial, rescue PCI resulted in lower rates of in-hospital death and the combined end point of death or heart failure at 1 year.[27] Similarly, the REACT (Rescue Angioplasty versus Conservative Treatment or Repeat Thrombolysis) trial found that event-free survival was higher in patients who received rescue PCI compared with their counterparts treated conservatively or with repeat fibrinolytic therapy.[28]

Fibrinolytic Agents

Four fibrinolytic agents have been developed and approved for use in STEMI (Table 2): streptokinase, alteplase, reteplase and tenecteplase (TNK)–tissue plasminogen activator (tPA). Streptokinase was the first developed thrombolytic agent, and acts on plasminogen, resulting in proteolytic activity on fibrin.[29] Importantly, streptokinase is derived from bacteria and nonselectively binds to plasminogen, and bleeding complications are higher. In the landmark GISSI trial, streptokinase showed a mortality benefit compared with placebo in STEMI.[33] Mortalities

were reduced 18% in the streptokinase recipients at 21 days (P = .0002, relative risk [RR], 0.81), and survival benefit seemed to be greater the earlier the therapy was given (RRs, 0.74, 0.80, 0.87, and 1.19 for the 0–3-h, 3–6-h, 6–9-h, and 9–12-h subgroups). One-year mortalities were also reduced, and this trial resulted in the widespread use of fibrinolytics in STEMI.

As recombinant t-PAs developed, subsequent studies were conducted to determine their use in the setting of STEMI. Alteplase was the first developed recombinant t-PA.[30] Alteplase has specificity for fibrin-bound plasminogen, which increases accuracy in targeting a thrombotic lesion and is less antigenic. In the landmark GUSTO-I (Global Utilization of Streptokinase and Tissue Plasminogen Activator for Occluded Coronary Arteries) trial, arterial patency at 90 minutes was observed to be highest in patients that received accelerated-dose tPA with heparin (81%), and mortalities were reduced at 1 year. (9.1% vs 10.1%; P<.05).[34] The GISSI-2 (GRUPPO ITALIANO PER LO STUDIO DELLA SOPRAVVIVENZA NELL'INFARTO MIOCARDICO) trial also confirmed a lower 6-month mortality in patients who received t-PA versus streptokinase (12.3% vs 11.7%; RR, 1.06; 95% CI, 0.97–1.15).[35]

As accelerated t-PA became preferred to streptokinase for STEMI, multiple trials were conducted to determine comparative efficacy of newer agents. Reteplase is a genetically modified t-PA similar to alteplase, but lacks the kringle 1 and epidermal growth factor domains responsible for rapid liver metabolization, which increases half-life.[31] The GUSTO-III trial assessed clinical outcomes of reteplase versus alteplase in 15,059 patients presenting with STEMI and found 30-day and 1-year mortalities were similar.[36,37]

In addition, TNK-tPA is a recombinant tissue plasminogen activator that has been extensively bioengineered to enhance the beneficial characteristics of alteplase. TNK-tPA has a 15-fold increased fibrin specificity with a significantly longer half-life and high arterial patency rates.[32,38] The ASSENT-2 trial compared TNK-tPA with alteplase and found almost identical 30-day mortalities (6.18% vs 6.15% respectively) with similar rates of intracerebral bleeding (0.93% vs 0.94%). However, TNK-tPA had fewer noncerebral bleeding events (26.43% vs 28.95%, P = .0003) and less need for blood transfusions (4.25 vs 5.49%, P = .0002).[39]

In a large network meta-analysis involving 40 clinical trials and 128,071 individuals receiving fibrinolytic agents for STEMI, a higher all-cause mortality in streptokinase (RR, 1.14 [95% CI,

Table 2
United States Food and Drug Administration–approved fibrinolytic therapies for ST-elevation myocardial infarction

Agent	Pharmacologic Properties	Intravenous Dosing	90-min TIMI 2 or 3 Flow Rates (%)	Clinical Comments
Streptokinase[7,29]	• Polypeptide derived from bacteria • Binds plasminogen nonspecifically	1.5 million units over 30–60 min	60–68	• Antigenic; risk of allergic reaction or anaphylaxis • Lower survival benefit compared with other agents • ICH rate ~0.4%–0.9%
Alteplase[7,30]	• Recombinant form of naturally occurring tPA (serine protease) • Fibrin specific	Up to 100 mg over 90 min	73–84	• Improved survival compared with streptokinase • Similar efficacy to other recombinant agents • Allergic reactions not common
Reteplase[7,31]	• Genetically modified recombinant plasminogen activator • Longer half-life than alteplase • Fibrin specific (less so than alteplase)	10 units over 2 min ×2 given 30 min apart	84	• Similar to other recombinant agents in terms of survival • Easy to administer given short infusion duration • Allergic reactions not common
Tenecteplase[7,32]	• Genetically bioengineered form of tPA • 15-fold higher fibrin specificity; long half-life	Weight based IV bolus: 30–50 mg	85	• Similar survival to other recombinant agents • Lower noncerebral major bleeding risk • Highly fibrin specific • Long half-life allowing bolus dosing

Abbreviations: ICH, intracranial hemorrhage; IV, intravenous; TIMI, Thrombolysis in Myocardial Infarction; tPA, tissue plasminogen activator.

1.05–1.24]) and nonaccelerated alteplase (RR, 1.26 [1·10–1·45]) infusions group was seen compared with accelerated alteplase, TNK-tPA, and reteplase infusions.[40] No mortality difference was seen between accelerated alteplase, TNK-tPA, and reteplase infusions. However, TNK-tPA was associated with a lower risk of major bleeding events (RR, 0.79 [95% CI 0.63–1.00]).

There is clear evidence to support that accelerated t-PA is preferred to streptokinase. Mortality outcomes are similar among alteplase, reteplase, and TNK-tPA, with some evidence suggesting that TNK-tPA may result in lower rates of major bleeding. In addition, TNK-tPA and reteplase are easier to administer. Clinicians should carefully assess whether any relative or absolute contraindications exist before using fibrinolytic therapy (Table 3).

Use of Concomitant Antithrombotic Therapies

Dual antiplatelet therapy (DAPT) is currently recommended with fibrinolytic treatment of STEMI.[7] Aspirin 162 to 325 mg should be given at presentation. In addition, clopidogrel loading is recommended at 300 mg, unless the patient is more than 75 years old (at which time, clopidogrel 75 mg daily is given without a load). In the CLARITY-TIMI (Clopidogrel as Adjunctive Reperfusion Therapy–Thrombolysis in Myocardial Infarction) 28 trial, improved arterial patency was seen in patients who received DAPT.[41] There is a paucity of data regarding the concomitant use of the newer $P2Y_{12}$ receptor inhibitors with fibrinolytic therapy after STEMI. In the TREAT (Ticagrelor in Patients With ST Elevation Myocardial Infarction Treated With Pharmacological Thrombolysis) trial, investigators found

Table 3
Contraindications to fibrinolytic therapy

Absolute Contraindications	Relative Contraindications
• Recent ICH • Structural cerebral vascular lesion • Intracranial neoplasm • Ischemic stroke <3 mo • Suspected aortic dissection • Active bleeding or bleeding disorder • Significant head injury <3 mo • Recent intracranial or spinal surgery • Severe uncontrolled hypertension	• History of severe poorly controlled hypertension • Hypertension at presentation (SBP >180 mm Hg or DBP >110 mm Hg) • Prolonged CPR or major surgery <3 wk • Prior ischemic stroke • Dementia • Internal bleeding past 2–4 wk • Noncompressible vascular puncture • Pregnancy • Active peptic ulcer • Current anticoagulant therapy with INR>1.7 or PT>15 s

Abbreviations: CPR, cardiopulmonary resuscitation; DBP, diastolic blood pressure; INR, International Normalized Ratio; PT, prothrombin time; SBP, systolic blood pressure.

that ticagrelor (180 mg loading followed by 90 mg twice daily) was noninferior to clopidogrel after fibrinolytic therapy.[42] At present, clopidogrel remains the antiplatelet of choice in patients receiving fibrinolytic therapy, but transition to ticagrelor or prasugrel may be considered, based predominantly on expert opinion, in patients with STEMI at 48 hours, especially those who have undergone PCI.

Background parenteral anticoagulant therapy is recommended in patients presenting with STEMI undergoing fibrinolytic therapy. A large meta-analysis found that the most superior regimens, with regard to mortality and bleeding, were alteplase, reteplase, and TNK in combination with anticoagulant therapy. Various therapeutic options exist, including unfractionated heparin (60-units/kg bolus followed by 12 units/kg/h), enoxaparin (30 mg intravenous [IV] plus 1 mg/kg subcutaneous), or fondaparinux (IV bolus followed by 2.5 mg subcutaneously 24 hours after bolus).

In addition, combination pharmacologic therapies have been studied, which includes the use of glycoprotein IIb/IIIa inhibitors given with half-dose fibrinolytic agents. The GUSTO-V trial showed similar outcomes in patients who received glycoprotein IIb/IIIa inhibitors with half-dose reteplase compared with full-dose reteplase; however, significantly higher bleeding rates were seen in the combination group.[43]

Complications

Complications of fibrinolytic therapy include major bleeding, stroke, and intracranial hemorrhage (ICH). ICH rates in most trials evaluating fibrinolytic agents are less than 1%.[44–46] ICH should be suspected in individuals who develop sudden neurologic changes, altered mental status, headache, vomiting, or a sudden blood pressure increase within 24 hours of fibrinolysis. Risk factors for ICH include older age (>65 years per Gurwitz and colleagues[46]), female sex, prior stroke, black ethnicity, systolic blood pressure of 140 mm Hg or more, diastolic blood pressure of 100 mm Hg or more, tPA dose more than 1.5 mg/kg, and a lower body weight (OR, 0.81 per 10-kg increase in body weight [CI, 0.76–0.87]).[44–46]

Major noncerebral bleeding events that can occur include gastrointestinal, genitourinary, and retroperitoneal bleeds. Major trials vary in how bleeding is reported, which leads to significant variation in bleeding rates depending on how the events were defined. Major bleeding rates reported with streptokinase are as high as 16% in some studies, but are typically 1% to 5%.[33,47] Alteplase has low rates of severe life-threatening bleeding at less than 1%.[36] Reteplase performs similarly, with major bleeding rates reported at 0.7% in the INJECT (International Joint Efficacy Comparison of Thrombolytics) trial.[48] In addition, TNK-tPA has been shown to have lower rates of bleeding that requires blood transfusion compared with alteplase, as reported in the ASSENT-1 trial (1.4% vs 7% respectively). Decreased major bleeding events were similarly observed with TNK-tPA in the ASSENT-2 trial.[49]

Streptokinase is unique given its antigenicity and hypotension or anaphylactic reactions are potential complications of therapy. In the GUSTO-1 trial, allergic and anaphylactic reactions were seen in 5.7% and 0.6% of patients respectively.[44] In a subsequent secondary analysis, no significant mortality difference was seen among those who experienced allergic side effects to streptokinase.[50]

Although the rates of stroke associated with fibrinolytic therapy are low, it remains associated with exceedingly high rates of morbidity and mortality. In GUSTO-I, of all strokes, 41% were fatal, 31% were disabling, and most (95%) occurred within 5 days of fibrinolytic therapy administration.[44]

FIBRINOLYTIC THERAPY IN SPECIFIC PATIENT POPULATIONS

Elderly Patients

Advanced age is a predictor of mortality, increased frequency of left ventricular free-wall rupture, major bleeding, and ICH after fibrinolysis. A national database analysis found that age greater than 75 years was associated with in-hospital mortality after multivariable analysis (OR, 5.95; 95% CI, 4.68–7.57).[51] In the STREAM (Strategic Reperfusion Early after Myocardial Infarction) trial, a 50% dose reduction of TNK in patients 75 years of age or older decreased the incidence of ICH with no overall change in outcomes. Clinicians must critically weigh the risks and benefits of fibrinolytic therapy in elderly individuals before initiating therapy and strongly consider PCI. Moreover, as previously mentioned, loading dose of clopidogrel is not recommended in patients more than 75 years of age.

Cardiogenic Shock

The evidence for fibrinolytic therapy in cardiogenic shock is limited.[52–54] Initial studies have shown no survival benefit, whereas small patient cohort results have been mixed comparing streptokinase with tissue plasminogen activator.[55] The GUSTO-1 trial observed no substantial mortality benefit between fibrinolytic strategies among the nearly 3000 included patients with cardiogenic shock.[56] In patients with cardiogenic shock, primary PCI has better clinical outcomes than fibrinolytic therapy. However, for patients who cannot receive timely primary PCI, fibrinolysis followed by urgent PCI (even if there is a delay of up to 24 hours) is the preferred management strategy.

Patients with Coronavirus Disease 2019

The pathogenesis of COVID-19 is associated with coagulopathy and abnormalities in the fibrinolytic system, which leads to a procoagulant state. There has been an emerging discussion of the utility of fibrinolytic therapy in the COVID-19 pandemic because of operational challenges related to PCI and COVID-19 transmission. Some experts have proposed the use of fibrinolytic therapy as part of a pharmacoinvasive strategy or primary reperfusion strategy in certain patients with COVID-19 infection presenting with STEMI. Interestingly, recent studies have shown that fibrinolytic therapy can improve survival in acute respiratory distress syndrome and may have a role in patients with COVID-19.[57,58] Such an approach reduces staff exposure risk and consumption of personal protective equipment. However, some suggest that fibrinolytic therapy in patients with COVID-19 with STEMI may be misguided, because fibrinolytic therapy remains an inferior reperfusion strategy compared with primary PCI in STEMI.[10,59] In addition, it is possible that a STEMI presentation may mimic other causes in COVID-19, such as myopericarditis, in which instances fibrinolytic therapy and invasive angiography may not be beneficial and may lead to unnecessary harm.[60]

SUMMARY

Fibrinolytic agents provide an important alternative therapeutic strategy in individuals presenting with STEMI. Ultimately, primary PCI is the preferred reperfusion strategy for most patients with STEMI, including elderly patients and patients with COVID-19 infection. Fibrinolytic therapy should always be considered when timely primary PCI cannot be delivered appropriately. Clinicians should promptly recognize the signs of fibrinolytic therapy failure and consider rescue PCI. When fibrinolytics are used, coronary angiography and revascularization should not be conducted within the initial 3 hours after fibrinolytic administration.

CLINICS CARE POINTS

- Fibrinolytic agents provide an important alternative therapeutic strategy in individuals presenting with ST-elevation myocardial infarction (STEMI).
- The effectiveness of fibrinolytic therapy is time sensitive, and best outcomes are noted within the initial 2 hours after symptom onset.
- Newer fibrinolytics more selectively target fibrin-bound plasminogen to reduce unintended off-target effects.
- Primary percutaneous coronary intervention (PCI) is the preferred reperfusion strategy for most patients with STEMI, including elderly patients and patients with coronavirus disease 2019 (COVID-19) infection.

- Fibrinolytic therapy should always be considered when timely primary PCI cannot be delivered appropriately.
- Prehospital fibrinolytic therapy administered by emergency medical services may improve outcomes and should be considered in the right clinical situation.
- The pharmacoinvasive approach of early routine PCI after fibrinolysis within 3 to 24 hours is currently recommended by major guidelines and has become the preferred strategy in many non–PCI-capable medical centers.
- Clinicians should promptly recognize the signs of fibrinolytic therapy failure and consider rescue PCI.
- Dual antiplatelet therapy (DAPT) is currently recommended with fibrinolytic treatment of STEMI.
- Complications of fibrinolytic therapy include major bleeding, stroke, and intracranial hemorrhage (ICH) with rates of ICH reported <1% in most trials.
- Clinicians must critically weigh the risks and benefits of fibrinolytic therapy in elderly individuals before initiating therapy due to higher complication rates (major bleed, ICH etc.).
- Fibrinolytic therapy in patients with COVID-19 with STEMI may be misguided if PCI is readily available because fibrinolytic therapy remains an inferior reperfusion strategy compared with primary PCI in STEMI. Ultimately, PCI remains the first-line intervention strategy in patient with COVID-19 presenting with STEMI if available.

REFERENCES

1. Kolodgie FD, Burke AP, Farb A, et al. The thin-cap fibroatheroma: a type of vulnerable plaque: the major precursor lesion to acute coronary syndromes. Curr Opin Cardiol 2001;16(5):285–92.
2. Scharf RE. Platelet signaling in primary haemostasis and arterial thrombus formation: part 1. Hamostaseologie 2018;38(4):203–10.
3. Knuttinen MG, Emmanuel N, Isa F, et al. Review of pharmacology and physiology in thrombolysis interventions. Semin Intervent Radiol 2010;27(4):374–83.
4. Kircher BJ, Topol EJ, O'Neill WW, et al. Prediction of infarct coronary artery recanalization after intravenous thrombolytic therapy. Am J Cardiol 1987;59(6):513–5.
5. Pasceri V, Andreotti F, Maseri A. Clinical markers of thrombolytic success. Eur Heart J 1996;17(Suppl E):35–41.
6. Mauri F, Maggioni AP, Franzosi MG, et al. A simple electrocardiographic predictor of the outcome of patients with acute myocardial infarction treated with a thrombolytic agent. A Gruppo Italiano per lo Studio della Sopravvivenza nell'Infarto Miocardico (GISSI-2)-Derived Analysis. J Am Coll Cardiol 1994;24(3):600–7.
7. O'Gara PT, Kushner FG, Ascheim DD, et al. 2013 ACCF/AHA guideline for the management of ST-elevation myocardial infarction: executive summary: a report of the American College of Cardiology Foundation/American Heart Association Task Force on Practice Guidelines. J Am Coll Cardiol 2013;61(4):485–510.
8. Ibanez B, James S, Agewall S, et al. 2017 ESC Guidelines for the management of acute myocardial infarction in patients presenting with ST-segment elevation: The Task Force for the management of acute myocardial infarction in patients presenting with ST-segment elevation of the European Society of Cardiology (ESC). Eur Heart J 2018;39(2):119–77.
9. Jneid H, Addison D, Bhatt DL, et al. 2017 AHA/ACC Clinical Performance and Quality Measures for Adults With ST-Elevation and Non-ST-Elevation Myocardial Infarction: A Report of the American College of Cardiology/American Heart Association Task Force on Performance Measures. J Am Coll Cardiol 2017;70(16):2048–90.
10. An international randomized trial comparing four thrombolytic strategies for acute myocardial infarction. N Engl J Med 1993;329(10):673–82.
11. Holmes DR Jr, Califf RM, Topol EJ. Lessons we have learned from the GUSTO trial. Global Utilization of Streptokinase and Tissue Plasminogen Activator for Occluded Arteries. J Am Coll Cardiol 1995;25(7 Suppl):10S–7S.
12. Boersma E, Maas AC, Deckers JW, et al. Early thrombolytic treatment in acute myocardial infarction: reappraisal of the golden hour. Lancet 1996;348(9030):771–5.
13. Weaver WD, Cerqueira M, Hallstrom AP, et al. Prehospital-initiated vs hospital-initiated thrombolytic therapy. The Myocardial Infarction Triage and Intervention Trial. JAMA 1993;270(10):1211–6.
14. Goldberg RJ, Mooradd M, Gurwitz JH, et al. Impact of time to treatment with tissue plasminogen activator on morbidity and mortality following acute myocardial infarction (The second National Registry of Myocardial Infarction). Am J Cardiol 1998;82(3):259–64.
15. Morrow DA, Antman EM, Sayah A, et al. Evaluation of the time saved by prehospital initiation of reteplase for ST-elevation myocardial infarction: results

of The Early Retavase-Thrombolysis in Myocardial Infarction (ER-TIMI) 19 trial. J Am Coll Cardiol 2002;40(1):71–7.

16. Danchin N, Blanchard D, Steg PG, et al. Impact of prehospital thrombolysis for acute myocardial infarction on 1-year outcome: results from the French Nationwide USIC 2000 Registry. Circulation 2004;110(14):1909–15.

17. Morrison LJ, Verbeek PR, McDonald AC, et al. Mortality and prehospital thrombolysis for acute myocardial infarction: A meta-analysis. JAMA 2000;283(20):2686–92.

18. Welsh RC, Travers A, Senaratne M, et al. Feasibility and applicability of paramedic-based prehospital fibrinolysis in a large North American center. Am Heart J 2006;152(6):1007–14.

19. Godfrey A, Borger J. EMS prehospital administration of thrombolytics for STEMI. [Updated 2020 Sep 27]. In: StatPearls [Internet]. Treasure Island (FL): StatPearls Publishing; 2021. Available at: https://www.ncbi.nlm.nih.gov/books/NBK545267/.

20. Vora AN, Holmes DN, Rokos I, et al. Fibrinolysis use among patients requiring interhospital transfer for ST-segment elevation myocardial infarction care: a report from the US National Cardiovascular Data Registry. JAMA Intern Med 2015;175(2): 207–15.

21. Antman EM, Anbe DT, Armstrong PW, et al. ACC/AHA guidelines for the management of patients with ST-elevation myocardial infarction–executive summary. A report of the American College of Cardiology/American Heart Association Task Force on Practice Guidelines (Writing Committee to revise the 1999 guidelines for the management of patients with acute myocardial infarction). J Am Coll Cardiol 2004;44(3):671–719.

22. Cantor WJ, Fitchett D, Borgundvaag B, et al. Routine early angioplasty after fibrinolysis for acute myocardial infarction. N Engl J Med 2009;360(26): 2705–18.

23. Borgia F, Goodman SG, Halvorsen S, et al. Early routine percutaneous coronary intervention after fibrinolysis vs. standard therapy in ST-segment elevation myocardial infarction: a meta-analysis. Eur Heart J 2010;31(17):2156–69.

24. Primary versus tenecteplase-facilitated percutaneous coronary intervention in patients with ST-segment elevation acute myocardial infarction (ASSENT-4 PCI): randomised trial. Lancet 2006; 367(9510):569–78.

25. Ellis SG, Tendera M, de Belder MA, et al. Facilitated PCI in patients with ST-elevation myocardial infarction. N Engl J Med 2008;358(21):2205–17.

26. Ross AM, Huber K, Zeymer U, et al. The impact of place of enrollment and delay to reperfusion on 90-day post-infarction mortality in the ASSENT-4 PCI trial: assessment of the safety and efficacy of a new treatment strategy with percutaneous coronary intervention. JACC Cardiovasc Interv 2009; 2(10):925–30.

27. Ellis SG, da Silva ER, Heyndrickx G, et al. Randomized comparison of rescue angioplasty with conservative management of patients with early failure of thrombolysis for acute anterior myocardial infarction. Circulation 1994;90(5):2280–4.

28. Gershlick AH, Stephens-Lloyd A, Hughes S, et al. Rescue angioplasty after failed thrombolytic therapy for acute myocardial infarction. N Engl J Med 2005;353(26):2758–68.

29. Capitanescu C, Macovei Oprescu AM, Ionita D, et al. Molecular processes in the streptokinase thrombolytic therapy. J Enzyme Inhib Med Chem 2016;31(6):1411–4.

30. Acheampong P, Ford GA. Pharmacokinetics of alteplase in the treatment of ischaemic stroke. Expert Opin Drug Metab Toxicol 2012;8(2):271–81.

31. Wooster MB, Luzier AB. Reteplase: a new thrombolytic for the treatment of acute myocardial infarction. Ann Pharmacother 1999;33(3):318–24.

32. Tanswell P, Modi N, Combs D, et al. Pharmacokinetics and pharmacodynamics of tenecteplase in fibrinolytic therapy of acute myocardial infarction. Clin Pharmacokinet 2002;41(15):1229–45.

33. Effectiveness of intravenous thrombolytic treatment in acute myocardial infarction. Gruppo Italiano per lo Studio della Streptochinasi nell'Infarto Miocardico (GISSI). Lancet 1986;1(8478):397–402.

34. The effects of tissue plasminogen activator, streptokinase, or both on coronary-artery patency, ventricular function, and survival after acute myocardial infarction. N Engl J Med 1993;329(22): 1615–22.

35. GISSI-2: a factorial randomised trial of alteplase versus streptokinase and heparin versus no heparin among 12,490 patients with acute myocardial infarction. Gruppo Italiano per lo Studio della Sopravvivenza nell'Infarto Miocardico. Lancet 1990;336(8707):65–71.

36. A comparison of reteplase with alteplase for acute myocardial infarction. N Engl J Med 1997;337(16): 1118–23.

37. Topol EJ, Ohman EM, Armstrong PW, et al. Survival outcomes 1 year after reperfusion therapy with either alteplase or reteplase for acute myocardial infarction: results from the Global Utilization of Streptokinase and t-PA for Occluded Coronary Arteries (GUSTO) III Trial. Circulation 2000;102(15): 1761–5.

38. Cannon CP, Gibson CM, McCabe CH, et al. TNK-tissue plasminogen activator compared with front-loaded alteplase in acute myocardial infarction: results of the TIMI 10B trial. Thrombolysis in Myocardial Infarction (TIMI) 10B Investigators. Circulation 1998;98(25):2805–14.

39. Van De Werf F, Adgey J, Ardissino D, et al. Single-bolus tenecteplase compared with front-loaded alteplase in acute myocardial infarction: the ASSENT-2 double-blind randomised trial. Lancet 1999;354(9180):716–22.

40. Jinatongthai P, Kongwatcharapong J, Foo CY, et al. Comparative efficacy and safety of reperfusion therapy with fibrinolytic agents in patients with ST-segment elevation myocardial infarction: a systematic review and network meta-analysis. Lancet 2017;390(10096):747–59.

41. Sabatine MS, Cannon CP, Gibson CM, et al. Addition of clopidogrel to aspirin and fibrinolytic therapy for myocardial infarction with ST-segment elevation. N Engl J Med 2005;352(12):1179–89.

42. Berwanger O, Nicolau JC, Carvalho AC, et al. Ticagrelor vs Clopidogrel After Fibrinolytic Therapy in Patients With ST-Elevation Myocardial Infarction: A Randomized Clinical Trial. JAMA Cardiol 2018; 3(5):391–9.

43. Topol EJ. Reperfusion therapy for acute myocardial infarction with fibrinolytic therapy or combination reduced fibrinolytic therapy and platelet glycoprotein IIb/IIIa inhibition: the GUSTO V randomised trial. Lancet 2001;357(9272):1905–14.

44. Gore JM, Granger CB, Simoons ML, et al. Stroke after thrombolysis. Mortality and functional outcomes in the GUSTO-I trial. Global Use of Strategies to Open Occluded Coronary Arteries. Circulation 1995;92(10):2811–8.

45. Huynh T, Cox JL, Massel D, et al. Predictors of intracranial hemorrhage with fibrinolytic therapy in unselected community patients: a report from the FASTRAK II project. Am Heart J 2004;148(1):86–91.

46. Gurwitz JH, Gore JM, Goldberg RJ, et al. Risk for intracranial hemorrhage after tissue plasminogen activator treatment for acute myocardial infarction. Participants in the National Registry of Myocardial Infarction 2. Ann Intern Med 1998; 129(8):597–604.

47. Randomised trial of intravenous streptokinase, oral aspirin, both, or neither among 17,187 cases of suspected acute myocardial infarction: ISIS-2. ISIS-2 (Second International Study of Infarct Survival) Collaborative Group. Lancet 1988;2(8607):349–60.

48. Randomised, double-blind comparison of reteplase double-bolus administration with streptokinase in acute myocardial infarction (INJECT): trial to investigate equivalence. International Joint Efficacy Comparison of Thrombolytics. Lancet 1995; 346(8971):329–36.

49. Van de Werf F, Cannon CP, Luyten A, et al. Safety assessment of single-bolus administration of TNK tissue-plasminogen activator in acute myocardial infarction: the ASSENT-1 trial. The ASSENT-1 Investigators. Am Heart J 1999;137(5):786–91.

50. Tsang TS, Califf RM, Stebbins AL, et al. Incidence and impact on outcome of streptokinase allergy in the GUSTO-I trial. Global Utilization of Streptokinase and t-PA in Occluded Coronary Arteries. Am J Cardiol 1997;79(9):1232–5.

51. Elbadawi A, Mahtta D, Elgendy IY, et al. Trends and Outcomes of Fibrinolytic Therapy for STEMI: Insights and Reflections in the COVID-19 Era. JACC Cardiovasc interventions 2020;13(19):2312–4.

52. Menon V, Hochman JS, Stebbins A, et al. Lack of progress in cardiogenic shock: lessons from the GUSTO trials. Eur Heart J 2000;21(23):1928–36.

53. Goldberg RJ, Gore JM, Alpert JS, et al. Cardiogenic shock after acute myocardial infarction. Incidence and mortality from a community-wide perspective, 1975 to 1988. N Engl J Med 1991; 325(16):1117–22.

54. Yusuf S, Collins R, Peto R, et al. Intravenous and intracoronary fibrinolytic therapy in acute myocardial infarction: overview of results on mortality, reinfarction and side-effects from 33 randomized controlled trials. Eur Heart J 1985;6(7):556–85.

55. Col NF, Gurwitz JH, Alpert JS, et al. Frequency of inclusion of patients with cardiogenic shock in trials of thrombolytic therapy. Am J Cardiol 1994;73(2): 149–57.

56. Holmes DR Jr, Bates ER, Kleiman NS, et al. Contemporary reperfusion therapy for cardiogenic shock: the GUSTO-I trial experience. The GUSTO-I Investigators. Global Utilization of Streptokinase and Tissue Plasminogen Activator for Occluded Coronary Arteries. J Am Coll Cardiol 1995;26(3): 668–74.

57. Liu C, Ma Y, Su Z, et al. Meta-Analysis of Preclinical Studies of Fibrinolytic Therapy for Acute Lung Injury. Front Immunol 2018;9:1898.

58. Wang J, Hajizadeh N, Moore EE, et al. Tissue plasminogen activator (tPA) treatment for COVID-19 associated acute respiratory distress syndrome (ARDS): A case series. J Thromb Haemost 2020; 18(7):1752–5.

59. Sudhakar D, Jneid H, Lakkis N, et al. Primary Percutaneous Coronary Intervention or Fibrinolytic Therapy in COVID 19 Patients Presenting With ST-Segment Elevation Myocardial Infarction. Am J Cardiol 2020;134:158.

60. Bangalore S, Sharma A, Slotwiner A, et al. ST-Segment Elevation in Patients with Covid-19 - A Case Series. N Engl J Med 2020;382(25): 2478–80.

Quality Improvement and Public Reporting in STEMI Care

Dan D. Nguyen, MD[a], Jacob A. Doll, MD[a,b],*

KEYWORDS

- STEMI • Quality improvement • Quality measures • Public reporting • Pay-for-performance

---

KEY POINTS

- Quality improvement interventions have led to substantial reductions in ischemic time for patients with ST-segment elevation myocardial infarction (STEMI).
- There are numerous quality and performance measures for STEMI; some are publicly reported, with mixed impact on patient outcomes.
- A multidisciplinary STEMI quality improvement program is recommended to analyze quality data, perform case reviews, and coordinate quality improvement interventions.

INTRODUCTION

Substantial progress has been made in the prevention and treatment of coronary artery disease (CAD), leading to a decades-long decline in mortality. The incidence of myocardial infarction (MI) also has declined; yet, more than 800,000 patients are hospitalized for an MI annually in the United States, approximately 1 every 40 seconds.[1] ST-segment elevation MI (STEMI) has been the focus of substantial efforts to optimize guideline-recommended medical therapies and reduce the time from symptom onset to coronary reperfusion. Despite the development of many novel drugs and interventions for this high-risk population, rates of in-hospital and 30-day mortality remain high.[2] In contrast with other encouraging trends of cardiovascular disease incidence and outcomes, mortality for STEMI patients has declined only modestly, if at all.[3,4]

There remains heterogeneity in STEMI care across the United States,[2] despite clear guidelines from professional societies supported by a strong evidence base.[5] Efforts to improve adherence to guideline-directed care are categorized broadly as quality improvement (QI). QI interventions may focus on recognizing and addressing quality gaps, redesigning care processes, or eliminating disparities related to race, gender, or other patient characteristics. Although all QI efforts ultimately seek improvement in clinical outcomes and quality of life, specific interventions may take many potential forms. One review proposed 9 distinct categories of interventions: (1) provider reminders; (2) facilitated relay of clinical data to providers; (3) audit and feedback; (4) provider education; (5) patient education; (6) promotion of self-monitoring; (7) patient reminders; (8) organizational change; and (9) financial, regulatory, or legislative incentives.[6] Given the diverse nature of QI interventions and heterogenous research methodologies, studies assessing STEMI QI interventions have been variable in terms of quality and generalizability.[7] Randomized controlled trials (RCTs) are rare. Some QI interventions, such as public reporting of outcomes, have had unanticipated adverse impacts on patient outcomes. This review, therefore, synthesizes and describes the most

---

[a] Division of Cardiology, Department of Medicine, University of Washington, 1959 NE Pacific Street, Seattle, WA 98195, USA; [b] VA Puget Sound Health Care System, 1660 S Columbian Way, Seattle, WA 98108, USA
* Corresponding author. VA Puget Sound Health Care System, 1660 S Columbian Way, S111-CARDIO, Seattle, WA 98108.
E-mail address: jdoll@uw.edu

Intervent Cardiol Clin 10 (2021) 391–400
https://doi.org/10.1016/j.iccl.2021.03.009
2211-7458/21/Published by Elsevier Inc.

effective QI interventions pertaining to STEMI care, summarizes quality measures for the assessment of STEMI care, and provides a framework for the development of a local STEMI QI program.

QUALITY IMPROVEMENT INITIATIVES ALONG THE STEMI CARE CONTINUUM

This section discusses QI initiatives that aim to improve STEMI care throughout athe patient's clinical course, from symptom onset to postdischarge follow-up (Fig. 1). The direct relationship between ischemic time and myocardial injury has been well established, so many STEMI QI efforts have focused on shortening the time to treatment, that is, the period from initial symptom onset to reperfusion with primary percutaneous coronary intervention (PCI) or thrombolytics.[8] Traditionally, efforts have focused on processes within the direct control of the hospital, such as door-to-device time. Hospitals also now look upstream, however, for opportunities to reduce ischemic time.

Symptom Onset to First Medical Contact

A prompt 9-1-1 call after the onset of STEMI symptoms may reduce ischemic time. Approximately 20% of Americans, however, are not aware of the 3 most common symptoms of MI; 6% of Americans are not aware of any of the symptoms of MI; and those without knowledge of any cardinal MI symptoms were 50% more likely to delay calling emergency medical services (EMS).[9] There have been no studies to date assessing the efficacy of QI interventions on improving symptom recognition, although several groups, including the US Centers for Disease Control and Prevention; National Heart, Lung, and Blood Institute; and American Heart Association (AHA), have sponsored national educational programs to raise symptom awareness. High-risk populations, such as women, racial and ethnic minorities, non-English speakers, and those with lower education levels may benefit the most from targeted, population-specific QI interventions.[10–12] Hospitals may coordinate with local public health and EMS agencies to encourage early recognition of MI symptoms and prompt EMS activation. This may be important particularly during the COVID-19 pandemic, when many patients may be reluctant to present to the hospital.[13]

First Medical Contact to Hospital

STEMI care frequently begins at first contact with EMS personnel. The portion of ischemic time from first medical contract to revascularization has been called first medical contact to balloon (FMC2B) time. EMS interventions that have been associated with shortened FMC2B times include: prehospital electrocardiogram (ECG) diagnosis; prehospital activation of the cardiac catheterization laboratory (CCL); bypass of non–PCI-capable hospitals; and bypass of the emergency department (ED) directly to the CCL.[14–16] These interventions cannot be performed solely by EMS personnel but instead require integration into local and regional hospital networks. Therefore, the AHA 2013 STEMI guidelines include a class I recommendation that "all communities should create and maintain a regional system of STEMI care that includes assessment and QI of EMS and hospital-based activities."[5]

Examples of successful regional STEMI care models include the AHA Mission: Lifeline program and the American College of Cardiology (ACC) Door-to-Balloon Alliance for Quality. These regional collaboratives do not focus solely on any 1 STEMI care process but instead bring together leadership within EMS and hospital systems to develop local, consensus-based protocols for EMS dispatch and transfer. These protocols are monitored through regular interdisciplinary meetings for collaborative quality

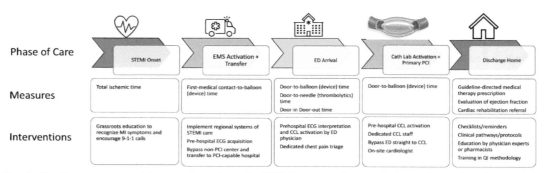

Fig. 1. Quality measures and interventions along the STEMI care continuum. Cath, cardiac catheterization; Lab, laboratory.

assessment and feedback.[17] Results of the Mission: Lifeline program at 5 years included increased use of prehospital ECGs (46% to 71%) and reductions in first medical contact to device times (93 minutes to 84 minutes). The proportion of patients presenting initially to PCI-capable centers via EMS improved from 38.4% to 43.0%.[3] In addition, state policies that mandate bypass of non–PCI-capable hospitals are associated with increased rates of achieving FMC2B time of less than 90 minutes.[18]

Door-to-Electrocardiogram Time

For patients whose first medical contact begins in the ED, immediate ECG acquisition, interpretation, and CCL activation can reduce delays in reperfusion. Several single-center studies have demonstrated significant reductions in door-to-ECG time with protocols for rapid identification and triage of chest pain patients.[19] ECG acquisition by nurse triage has been shown to increase the number of patients undergoing ECG within 10 minutes by approximately 10%.[20,21] Once obtained, an ECG must be interpreted correctly by a clinician with the ability to activate the CCL. In a nonrandomized, quasi-experimental study, ECG review by an interventional cardiologist was facilitated by sending a scanned ECG to a cardiologist's cellular phone, associated with a 39-minute improvement in door-to-balloon (D2B) time.[22] Additional time savings may be achieved by allowing ED clinicians to interpret the ECG and activate the CCL.[7,23]

Door-to-Balloon Time

A D2B time, also referred to as door-to-device time, of less than 90 minutes remains an important marker of STEMI care quality, despite increasing focus on more holistic measures of ischemic time. Shorter D2B times are associated with smaller infarct size and lower mortality rates.[24,25] D2B time has featured prominently in public reporting and pay-for-performance interventions by the Centers for Medicare & Medicaid Services (CMS), resulting in substantial incentives to optimize local care processes.

Seminal work by Bradley and colleagues[14] in 2006 demonstrated marked variability in hospital D2B times. A survey of 365 hospitals identified 6 factors that were independently associated with shorter times:

1. Allowing ED physicians to activate the CCL, rather than a cardiologist
2. Developing a centralized paging system to activate the CCL in 1 call

3. Prehospital activation of the CCL by ED clinician
4. Rapid CCL staff arrival
5. Having an attending cardiologist on site at all times
6. Real-time feedback and communication between ED and cardiology staff

Subsequent observational studies have supported these interventions, demonstrating D2B time reductions with a regional hub-and-spoke hospital model with electronic transmission of ECGs (5–39 min reduction),[22,26] ED activation of CCL[27] (38-min reduction), and a care pathway with electronic ECG transmission and bypassing the ED with feedback aimed at reducing ED to CCL handoff time.[28] In the United States, there has been a marked reduction in D2B times since the advent of D2B public reporting in 2005, undoubtedly due to the adaptation of these best practices to local circumstances at thousands of hospitals. This represents one of the most successful large-scale QI campaigns in the history of cardiovascular medicine.

RCTs of QI interventions have yielded less impressive impacts on D2B time, with various multicomponent QI strategies (including audit and feedback, clinical pathways, and performance assessment) showing modest or no improvement.[29–31] It is possible that QI efforts have hit a ceiling, with diminishing returns for additional efforts at time saving. In addition, the impact of reduced D2B times on patient outcomes still is debated,[32,33] and some studies caution that efforts to optimize D2B times can be costly, resulting in frequent false activations and clinician burnout.[34] Nonetheless, hospitals are encouraged to maintain and improve clinical systems focused on D2B time. In addition, there are ongoing efforts to further optimize this process, including algorithms for EMS interpretation of prehospital ECGs to reduce false-positive and false-negative CCL activations.[35]

Door-in Door-out Time

For patients transferred via EMS or private vehicle to a non–PCI-capable center, the AHA/ACC Task Force on Performance Measures recommends a door-in door-out (DIDO) time (ie, the time from patient presentation to patient leaving the ED in transfer to a PCI-capable center) of less than 30 minutes.[36] Yet, Herrin and colleagues[37] demonstrated that only 10% of patients achieved this standard. Some barriers to achieving this metric are similar to challenges facing FMC2B time optimization: a fragmented health care system, with each hospital operating independently; poor communication between hospitals and EMS services; and heterogenous hospital triage and transfer processes. Moreover, 9-1-1 operators typically prioritize field activations over transfer calls, necessitating specific protocols with local EMS providers for interhospital STEMI transfers.

Regional QI interventions focused broadly on ischemia time reduction have shown improved DIDO times for hospitals without primary PCI facilities. These QI interventions were multifaceted and included protocolized prehospital treatment algorithms for referring hospitals, tracking of quality-assurance measures with frequent feedback, and establishing a network for outcomes data collection and analysis for rural hospitals.[38,39] In addition, specific system factors that appear to improve DIDO time include EMS transport to hospital rather than personal transport, prehospital ECG acquisition, and statewide QI leadership for STEMI QI.[40,41]

Door-to-Needle Time

When FMC2B time is anticipated to be greater than 120 minutes, fibrinolytic therapy may be the preferred reperfusion strategy, and guidelines recommend fibrinolytic therapy be administered within 30 minutes of hospital arrival.[5] Because primary PCI has increased and fibrinolytic therapy use has decreased over the past 2 decades, there have been concurrent increases in door-to-needle time for non-PCI patients, highlighting the need for ongoing QI.[42]

A meta-analysis by McDermott and colleagues[35] showed that door-to-needle time decreased with policy changes, allowing for fibrinolytics to be administered in the ED rather than in the cardiac care unit, fast-tracking pathways for direct–to–critical care unit admission from EMS, and training of ED nurses to administer fibrinolytic therapy. Currently, EMS and hospital protocols are recommended for the administration of fibrinolysis when PCI is not possible or when transfer times are prohibitive.[39]

In-Hospital and Postdischarge Care

After reperfusion (if possible), continuation of optimal STEMI care involves in-hospital and post-discharge delivery of appropriate therapies. The benefits of secondary prevention have been reviewed extensively elsewhere.[5] Rates of guideline-directed medical therapy prescribed during MI hospitalization, however, remain suboptimal, with only 80% of patients receiving all appropriate medications at the time of discharge for MI.[2]

Several QI interventions have improved the prescription of secondary prevention

medications. Broadly, these interventions involve multidisciplinary collaboration and/or use of clinical care pathways to improve guideline-adherent care. A systematic review by Bahiru and colleagues[43] identified 8 RCTs that demonstrated a 0% to 15.2% increased use of in-hospital therapies, and 11 RCTs demonstrating a 0% to 7.2% increase in guideline-directed therapies at discharge. Examples of successful QI interventions included "academic detailing" by pharmacists,[43] education of hospital administration by physician experts,[44] checklists and reminders,[45] clinical pathways,[33] and training hospital leadership in QI process.[46]

Hospitals increasingly are responsible for postdischarge patient care, to optimize outcomes and reduce costly readmissions. Guideline-recommended postdischarge care elements include lifestyle modification, medication adherence, management of existing comorbidities, early follow-up, and enrollment in cardiac rehabilitation (CR).[5] CR reduces post-MI mortality and is an effective method of delivering patient education and encouraging medication adherence. Despite this benefit, CR enrollment and completion are low. Multiple strategies have been tested to improve participation, including motivational invitations based on behavior theory or social-cognitive theory, structured outreach, home visits, peer navigation, and home-based CR. In a systematic review, Pio and colleagues[47] demonstrated that face-to-face enrollment invitation from nurses or allied health professionals was the most successful enrollment intervention and home-based CR was most successful at CR retention.

Although early follow-up and care continuity intuitively may seem beneficial, data supporting any specific follow-up strategy are lacking. Very early follow-up within 7 days of MI was not associated with improved mortality, in contrast with data regarding hospitalized heart failure patients.[48] Advanced practice providers and physicians may be equally effective in delivering postdischarge care.[49] In the absence of compelling evidence, guideline recommendations to "facilitate effective, coordinated outpatient care for all patients with STEMI" may be adapted to the local environment.[5]

DISCUSSION: MONITORING QUALITY IMPROVEMENT PROCESSES AND OUTCOMES

Hospitals should develop data-driven systems for monitoring STEMI care and assessing the impact of QI interventions. Although other QI interventions may dissolve after achieving a pre-specified goal, a permanent STEMI QI infrastructure may be required to meet current and future care priorities. In many hospitals, this may be an extension of ongoing efforts to reduce D2B times or avoid readmissions. Mission: Lifeline STEMI program standards recommend, for example, that each hospital form a multidisciplinary team that meets regularly to make continuous quality care improvements. Whether or not hospitals actively engage in QI for STEMI, there are multiple quality measures for MI that are publicly reported and influence payments from the CMS.

Quality Measure Reporting
MI care long has been a focus of public reporting and pay-for-performance interventions. Acute MI 30-day mortality and readmissions are reported on the CMS Hospital Compare Web site and influence hospital payments via the Hospital Value-Based Purchasing (VBP) Program and Hospital Readmissions Reduction Program. Although the impact of these financial interventions on STEMI care and outcomes has not been characterized definitively,[50] inclusion of MI process and outcomes measures in VBP programs undoubtedly have stimulated local QI efforts and infrastructure. As an example, D2B time once was a focus of the CMS VBP program; significant improvements over the past 15 years have resulted in its retirement from the VBP calculation.

In addition, the ACC/AHA Task Force on Performance Measures identified other MI quality measures in consensus documents published in 2008 and 2017. The 2017 ACC/AHA STEMI/non-STEMI Measure Set includes 24 measures that are evidenced-based, modifiable, and clinically impactful.[51] These measures encompass 4 categories: effective clinical care, communication and care coordination, patient safety, and population-based health. Hospitals are advised to examine both the publicly reported CMS outcomes and these process measures when considering holistic STEMI program performance.

Clinical Registries
In parallel with federal efforts to measure and report MI care quality, clinical societies have developed registries to provide member hospitals with feedback on quality measures and benchmarking with peer institutions. Three US QI registries currently exist for patients with MI/STEMI: ACC/National Cardiovascular Data Registry (NCDR) Chest Pain–MI registry; ACC/NCDR CathPCI registry; and AHA Get With The Guidelines (GWTG)–Coronary Artery Disease registry. Measuring the impact of clinical registries on care quality has been challenging; participating hospitals may have superior processes of care relative to nonparticipating hospitals, but it is unclear if this can be attributed solely to the registry.[52] Registries may offer diverse, and difficult to quantify, support for QI efforts. For example, membership with the AHA GWTG registry includes reporting of outcomes data to hospital leadership but also feedback from AHA QI experts, collaborative learning sessions, hospital tool kits, and hospital recognition as a high-quality STEMI center. Overall, performance on key ACC/AHA process measures has improved over time among registry participants.[2]

Local Quality Improvement Programs
Although regional and national programs may provide important infrastructure for data acquisition and reporting, STEMI QI interventions ultimately must be implemented at the local level. Prior research has identified 8 themes of successful STEMI QI programs, using D2B time interventions as a model: (1) commitment to an explicit goal; (2) senior management support; (3) innovative protocols; (4) flexibility in refining protocols; (5) uncompromising leadership; (6) collaborative teams; (7) data feedback to monitor progress; and (8) an organizational culture that fosters resilience.[53] These aspirational QI characteristics may be best organized as a standing, multidisciplinary team that meets regularly to analyze STEMI data (from local or national registry sources), perform case review, and coordinate QI interventions.

Best practices for this type of collaborative QI effort have not been defined explicitly, but it is reasonable to learn from analogous processes, such as morbidity and mortality (M&M) conferences and root cause analysis (RCA). M&M conferences were pioneered by the surgical and anesthesiology communities but now have become widespread among most specialties in medicine. Traditionally, M&M serves as a platform to explore the patient, provider, and institutional factors that contribute to error in a collaborative, nonjudgmental fashion, so that performance and system factors can be improved. Several factors contribute to a successful M&M conference, including careful and diverse case selection; participation by fellows-in-training, faculty, ancillary staff, and members of multidisciplinary care team when applicable; audience participation; employment of cause-and-effect diagrams for system improvement efforts; review of

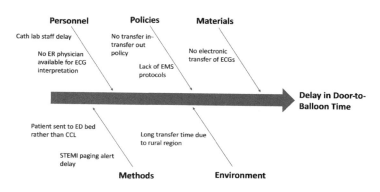

Fig. 2. Example of an RCA examining potential factors leading to prolonged FMC2B time. Cath, cardiac catheterization; ER, emergency room; Lab, laboratory.

guidelines to promote education; and conclusion with potential action items to improve quality of care provided.[54] As applied to STEMI care, an M&M framework may be applied to cases that do not meet quality standards, including delayed FMC2B time or poor patient outcomes.

Similarly, RCA is a systematic process for identifying underlying causes for problems and an approach for responding to them (Fig. 2). Unlike M&M conferences, which emphasize collaborative and open discussion, RCA may be a targeted tool for investigating systems issues, often implemented by a small team with appropriate clinical expertise.[55] For instance, 1 hospital STEMI program reviewed all 25 patient deaths over a 5-year period, noted 8 potentially preventable deaths, and identified prolonged ischemia time as a critical factor in poor outcomes.[56]

Once a care gap is identified, interventions to improve quality may be organized around 1 of several evidence-based QI frameworks, including Plan-Do-Study-Act (PDSA), Six Sigma, and Lean. Each of these approaches emphasizes iterative cycles of goal setting, data analysis, planning, implementation, and monitoring.[57] When used appropriately, these tools assist teams in applying evidence-based practices to diverse local environment[58] (Fig. 3).

Public Reporting

Public reporting of care processes and patient outcomes is intended to assist individuals in making informed decisions when choosing a health care provider and to benchmark hospitals and physicians to incentivize QI. These programs have been the subject of controversy since their inception in the 1990s. Reporting of MI outcomes by the CMS Hospital Compare program has been associated with reductions in 30-day mortality and readmission rates.[59] But other studies have noted that these improvements may reflect only secular trends present prior to public reporting and that hospital-level process measures explained little of the observed differences in mortality.[60,61]

Of particular importance to STEMI care, public reporting of PCI and coronary artery bypass graft mortality is present in several states. Public reporting of PCI mortality in New York, Pennsylvania, and Massachusetts was associated with lower in-hospital and 6-month mortality compared with

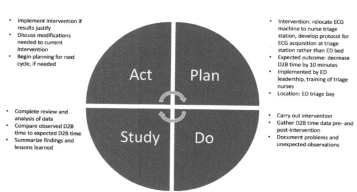

Fig. 3. Example of a PDSA QI cycle focused on reducing D2B time by shortening time to first ECG among patients with chest pain.

states without mandatory public reporting, despite similar estimated procedural risk.[62] These same states, however, also had significantly lower use of PCI for patients with MI, potential evidence for risk-averse case selection.[63] In New York State, public reporting was associated with a reduction in PCI rates for patients with out-of-hospital cardiac arrest and patients with cardiogenic shock.[64] Patients with MI had 21% higher odds of in-hospital mortality in public reporting states compared with non–public-reporting states, driven primarily by more high-risk patients not undergoing revascularization in public-reporting states.[65] Physicians are mistrustful of public reporting of PCI outcomes and admit to risk-averse case selection.[66,67] Finally, public reporting has not been widely used by patients in choosing physicians.[66] In total, the evidence suggests that public reporting of PCI outcomes may have some benefit for patients who receive PCI but overall is associated with worse MI outcomes due to avoidance of PCI for those high-risk patients who may benefit most.

Alternatively, a collaborative, nonpublic method of quality benchmarking may be considered. In 1997, the Blue Cross Blue Shield of Michigan Cardiovascular Consortium implemented a registry-based collaboration between PCI hospitals that focused on quality measure reporting and shared best practices. Compared with New York, Michigan had less risk averse case selection, although slightly worse risk-adjusted mortality.[68]

Although public reporting theoretically is a powerful tool for encouraging improved care processes, in practice it has been associated with adverse impacts on case selection and MI outcomes. It remains to be seen if and how public reporting will have an impact on STEMI care in the future. Potential areas for future policy innovation and research include developing risk-adjustment models or case exclusion criteria to avoid risk-avoidant behavior; transitioning from procedure-based (eg, PCI) quality measurement to disease-based (eg, MI) registries; and preferential reporting of modifiable process measures rather than outcomes.[69]

CLINICS CARE POINTS

Significant advances have been made in improving systems of care for patients with STEMI through QI initiatives at the local, regional, and national levels. For a hospital seeking to develop or improve its STEMI QI

program, it is challenging to recommend specific interventions that will be universally effective. Resources and barriers vary from hospital to hospital. Although STEMI best practices are supported by a strong base of high-quality evidence, the evidence describing QI interventions is of lower quality, and not all QI interventions have resulted in improved outcomes. Nonetheless, several themes have emerged from the literature, and the authors recommend the following components of a holistic STEMI QI program:

- Participation in a regional collaborative for STEMI care, including regular communication and feedback with EMS services
- Participation in an MI registry, or alternative mechanism to obtain MI process and quality measures
- Supporting a local multidisciplinary team to regularly review STEMI processes and outcomes
- Performing case review of adverse outcomes
- Implementing routine QI interventions using PDSA, Six Sigma, or Lean methodology

This QI infrastructure, supported by dedicated leadership and grounded in high-quality data, will ensure hospitals are well equipped to address current and future challenges for STEMI patients.

DISCLOSURE

The authors have nothing to disclose.

REFERENCES

1. Virani SS, Alonso A, Benjamin EJ, et al. Heart Disease and Stroke Statistics-2020 Update: A Report From the American Heart Association. Circulation 2020;141(9):e139–596.
2. Masoudi FA, Ponirakis A, de Lemos JA, et al. Trends in U.S. Cardiovascular Care: 2016 Report From 4 ACC National Cardiovascular Data Registries. J Am Coll Cardiol 2017;69(11):1427–50.
3. Granger CB, Bates ER, Jollis JG, et al. Improving Care of STEMI in the United States 2008 to 2012. J Am Heart Assoc 2019;8(1):e008096.
4. Sugiyama T, Hasegawa K, Kobayashi Y, et al. Differential time trends of outcomes and costs of care for acute myocardial infarction hospitalizations by ST elevation and type of intervention in the United States, 2001-2011. J Am Heart Assoc 2015;4(3):e001445.
5. O'Gara PT, Kushner FG, Ascheim DD, et al. 2013 ACCF/AHA guideline for the management of ST-

elevation myocardial infarction: a report of the American College of Cardiology Foundation/American Heart Association Task Force on Practice Guidelines. Circulation 2013;127(4):e362–425.

6. Bravata DM, Sundaram V, Lewis R, et al. Closing the Quality Gap: A Critical Analysis of Quality Improvement Strategies (Vol 5: Asthma Care). Rockville (MD): Agency for Healthcare Research and Quality (US).

7. Camp-Rogers T, Kurz MC, Brady WJ. Hospital-based strategies contributing to percutaneous coronary intervention time reduction in the patient with ST-segment elevation myocardial infarction: a review of the "system-of-care" approach. Am J Emerg Med 2012;30(3):491–8.

8. Bates ER, Jacobs AK. Time to treatment in patients with STEMI. N Engl J Med 2013;369(10):889–92.

9. Mahajan S, Valero-Elizondo J, Khera R, et al. Variation and disparities in awareness of myocardial infarction symptoms among adults in the United States. JAMA Netw open 2019;2(12):e1917885.

10. Lichtman JH, Leifheit-Limson EC, Watanabe E, et al. Symptom recognition and healthcare experiences of young women with acute myocardial infarction. Circ Cardiovasc Qual Outcomes 2015; 8(2 Suppl 1):S31–8.

11. Nguyen HL, Saczynski JS, Gore JM, et al. Age and sex differences in duration of prehospital delay in patients with acute myocardial infarction: a systematic review. Circ Cardiovasc Qual Outcomes 2010; 3(1):82–92.

12. Hand M, Brown C, Horan M, et al. The national heart attack alert program: progress at 5 years in educating providers, patients, and the public and future directions. J Thromb Thrombolysis 1998; 6(1):9–17.

13. Shah K, Tang D, Ibrahim F, et al. Surge in Delayed Myocardial Infarction Presentations: An Inadvertent Consequence of Social Distancing During the COVID-19 Pandemic. JACC Case Rep 2020;2(10): 1642–7.

14. Bradley EH, Herrin J, Wang Y, et al. Strategies for reducing the door-to-balloon time in acute myocardial infarction. N Engl J Med 2006;355(22):2308–20.

15. Anderson LL, French WJ, Peng SA, et al. Direct transfer from the referring hospitals to the catheterization laboratory to minimize reperfusion delays for primary percutaneous coronary intervention: insights from the national cardiovascular data registry. Circ Cardiovasc Interv 2015;8(9):e002477.

16. Fosbol EL, Granger CB, Jollis JG, et al. The impact of a statewide pre-hospital STEMI strategy to bypass hospitals without percutaneous coronary intervention capability on treatment times. Circulation 2013;127(5):604–12.

17. Bagai A, Al-Khalidi HR, Sherwood MW, et al. Regional systems of care demonstration project: Mission: Lifeline STEMI Systems Accelerator: design and methodology. Am Heart J 2014;167(1):15–21.e13.

18. Green JL, Jacobs AK, Holmes D, et al. Taking the Reins on Systems of Care for ST-segment-elevation myocardial infarction patients: a report from the american heart association mission: lifeline program. Circ Cardiovasc Interv 2018;11(5):e005706.

19. Phelan MP, Glauser J, Smith E, et al. Improving emergency department door-to-electrocardiogram time in ST segment elevation myocardial infarction. Crit Pathw Cardiol 2009;8(3):119–21.

20. Lee CK, Meng SW, Lee MH, et al. The impact of door-to-electrocardiogram time on door-to-balloon time after achieving the guideline-recommended target rate. PLoS One 2019;14(9): e0222019.

21. Scott IA, Denaro CP, Hickey AC, et al. Optimising care of acute coronary syndromes in three Australian hospitals. Int J Qual Health Care 2004;16(4): 275–84.

22. Chen KC, Yen DH, Chen CD, et al. Effect of emergency department in-hospital tele-electrocardiographic triage and interventional cardiologist activation of the infarct team on door-to-balloon times in ST-segment-elevation acute myocardial infarction. Am J Cardiol 2011;107(10):1430–5.

23. Bradley EH, Nallamothu BK, Curtis JP, et al. Summary of evidence regarding hospital strategies to reduce door-to-balloon times for patients with ST-segment elevation myocardial infarction undergoing primary percutaneous coronary intervention. Crit Pathw Cardiol 2007;6(3):91–7.

24. Guerchicoff A, Brener SJ, Maehara A, et al. Impact of delay to reperfusion on reperfusion success, infarct size, and clinical outcomes in patients with ST-segment elevation myocardial infarction: the INFUSE-AMI Trial (INFUSE-Anterior Myocardial Infarction). JACC Cardiovasc Interv 2014;7(7): 733–40.

25. Cannon CP, Gibson CM, Lambrew CT, et al. Relationship of symptom-onset-to-balloon time and door-to-balloon time with mortality in patients undergoing angioplasty for acute myocardial infarction. JAMA 2000;283(22):2941–7.

26. Alexander T, Mullasari AS, Joseph G, et al. A System of Care for Patients With ST-Segment Elevation Myocardial Infarction in India: The Tamil Nadu-ST-Segment Elevation Myocardial Infarction Program. JAMA Cardiol 2017;2(5):498–505.

27. Khot UN, Johnson ML, Ramsey C, et al. Emergency department physician activation of the catheterization laboratory and immediate transfer to an immediately available catheterization laboratory reduce door-to-balloon time in ST-elevation myocardial infarction. Circulation 2007;116(1):67–76.

28. Scholz KH, Maier SK, Jung J, et al. Reduction in treatment times through formalized data feedback:

results from a prospective multicenter study of ST-segment elevation myocardial infarction. JACC Cardiovasc Interv 2012;5(8):848–57.

29. Lytle BL, Li S, Lofthus DM, et al. Targeted versus standard feedback: results from a randomized quality improvement trial. Am Heart J 2015;169(1):132–41.e2.

30. Huffman MD, Mohanan PP, Devarajan R, et al. Effect of a quality improvement intervention on clinical outcomes in patients in india with acute myocardial infarction: the ACS QUIK randomized clinical trial. JAMA 2018;319(6):567–78.

31. Wu Y, Li S, Patel A, et al. Effect of a quality of care improvement initiative in patients with acute coronary syndrome in resource-constrained hospitals in china: a randomized clinical trial. JAMA Cardiol 2019;4(5):418–27.

32. Nallamothu BK, Normand SL, Wang Y, et al. Relation between door-to-balloon times and mortality after primary percutaneous coronary intervention over time: a retrospective study. Lancet 2015;385(9973):1114–22.

33. Menees DS, Peterson ED, Wang Y, et al. Door-to-balloon time and mortality among patients undergoing primary PCI. N Engl J Med 2013;369(10):901–9.

34. Lange DC, Conte S, Pappas-Block E, et al. Cancellation of the Cardiac Catheterization Lab After Activation for ST-segment-elevation myocardial infarction. Circ Cardiovasc Qual Outcomes 2018;11(8):e004464.

35. McDermott KA, Helfrich CD, Sales AE, et al. A review of interventions and system changes to improve time to reperfusion for ST-segment elevation myocardial infarction. J Gen Intern Med 2008;23(8):1246–56.

36. Krumholz HM, Anderson JL, Bachelder BL, et al. ACC/AHA 2008 performance measures for adults with ST-elevation and non-ST-elevation myocardial infarction: a report of the American College of Cardiology/American Heart Association Task Force on Performance Measures (Writing Committee to Develop Performance Measures for ST-Elevation and Non-ST-Elevation Myocardial Infarction) Developed in Collaboration With the American Academy of Family Physicians and American College of Emergency Physicians Endorsed by the American Association of Cardiovascular and Pulmonary Rehabilitation, Society for Cardiovascular Angiography and Interventions, and Society of Hospital Medicine. J Am Coll Cardiol 2008;52(24):2046–99.

37. Herrin J, Miller LE, Turkmani DF, et al. National performance on door-in to door-out time among patients transferred for primary percutaneous coronary intervention. Arch Intern Med 2011;171(21):1879–86.

38. Henry TD, Unger BT, Sharkey SW, et al. Design of a standardized system for transfer of patients with ST-elevation myocardial infarction for percutaneous coronary intervention. Am Heart J 2005;150(3):373–84.

39. Jollis JG, Mehta RH, Roettig ML, et al. Reperfusion of acute myocardial infarction in North Carolina emergency departments (RACE): study design. Am Heart J 2006;152(5):851.e1-11.

40. Mumma BE, Eggert J, Mahler SA, et al. Association Between Hospital Practices and Door-in-door-out Time in ST-segment Elevation Myocardial Infarction. Crit Pathw Cardiol 2016;15(4):165–8.

41. Shi O, Khan AM, Rezai MR, et al. Factors associated with door-in to door-out delays among ST-segment elevation myocardial infarction (STEMI) patients transferred for primary percutaneous coronary intervention: a population-based cohort study in Ontario, Canada. BMC Cardiovasc Disord 2018;18(1):204.

42. Hira RS, Bhatt DL, Fonarow GC, et al. Temporal trends in care and outcomes of patients receiving fibrinolytic therapy compared to primary percutaneous coronary intervention: insights from the get with the guidelines coronary artery disease (GWTG-CAD) Registry. J Am Heart Assoc 2016;5(10):e004113.

43. Bahiru E, Agarwal A, Berendsen MA, et al. Hospital-based quality improvement interventions for patients with acute coronary syndrome: a systematic review. Circ Cardiovasc Qual Outcomes 2019;12(9):e005513.

44. Berner ES, Baker CS, Funkhouser E, et al. Do local opinion leaders augment hospital quality improvement efforts? A randomized trial to promote adherence to unstable angina guidelines. Med Care 2003;41(3):420–31.

45. Berwanger O, Guimarães HP, Laranjeira LN, et al. Effect of a multifaceted intervention on use of evidence-based therapies in patients with acute coronary syndromes in Brazil: the BRIDGE-ACS randomized trial. JAMA 2012;307(19):2041–9.

46. Flather MD, Babalis D, Booth J, et al. Cluster-randomized trial to evaluate the effects of a quality improvement program on management of non-ST-elevation acute coronary syndromes: The European Quality Improvement Programme for Acute Coronary Syndromes (EQUIP-ACS). Am Heart J 2011;162(4):700–7.e1.

47. Pio CSA, Chaves G, Davies P, et al. Interventions to promote patient utilization of cardiac rehabilitation: cochrane systematic review and meta-analysis. J Clin Med 2019;8(2):189.

48. Hess CN, Shah BR, Peng SA, et al. Association of early physician follow-up and 30-day readmission after non-ST-segment-elevation myocardial infarction among older patients. Circulation 2013;128(11):1206–13.

49. Rymer JA, Chen AY, Thomas L, et al. Advanced Practice Provider Versus Physician-Only Outpatient

Follow-Up After Acute Myocardial Infarction. J Am Heart Assoc 2018;7(17):e008481.

50. Chatterjee P, Joynt KE. Do cardiology quality measures actually improve patient outcomes? J Am Heart Assoc 2014;3(1):e000404.

51. Jneid H, Addison D, Bhatt DL, et al. 2017 AHA/ACC Clinical Performance and Quality Measures for Adults With ST-Elevation and Non-ST-Elevation Myocardial Infarction: A Report of the American College of Cardiology/American Heart Association Task Force on Performance Measures. J Am Coll Cardiol 2017;70(16):2048–90.

52. Heidenreich PA, Hernandez AF, Yancy CW, et al. Get With The Guidelines program participation, process of care, and outcome for Medicare patients hospitalized with heart failure. Circ Cardiovasc Qual Outcomes 2012;5(1):37–43.

53. Bradley EH, Curry LA, Webster TR, et al. Achieving rapid door-to-balloon times: how top hospitals improve complex clinical systems. Circulation 2006;113(8):1079–85.

54. McNamara DA, Hall HM, Hardin EA. Rethinking the modern cardiology morbidity and mortality conference: harmonizing quality improvement and education. J Am Coll Cardiol 2019;73(7):868–72.

55. Charles R, Hood B, Derosier JM, et al. How to perform a root cause analysis for workup and future prevention of medical errors: a review. Patient Saf Surg 2016;10:20.

56. El Sakr F, Kenaan M, Menees D, et al. Root Cause Analysis of Deaths in ST-Segment Elevation Myocardial Infarctions Treated With Primary PCI: What Can We Do Better? J Invasive Cardiol 2017;29(5):164–8.

57. Silver SA, Harel Z, McQuillan R, et al. How to Begin a Quality Improvement Project. Clin J Am Soc Nephrol 2016;11(5):893–900.

58. Kelly EW, Kelly JD, Hiestand B, et al. Six Sigma process utilization in reducing door-to-balloon time at a single academic tertiary care center. Prog Cardiovasc Dis 2010;53(3):219–26.

59. Werner RM, Bradlow ET. Public reporting on hospital process improvements is linked to better patient outcomes. Health Aff (Millwood) 2010;29(7):1319–24.

60. Bradley EH, Herrin J, Elbel B, et al. Hospital quality for acute myocardial infarction: correlation among process measures and relationship with short-term mortality. JAMA 2006;296(1):72–8.

61. Ryan AM, Nallamothu BK, Dimick JB. Medicare's public reporting initiative on hospital quality had modest or no impact on mortality from three key conditions. Health Aff (Millwood) 2012;31(3):585–92.

62. Cavender MA, Joynt KE, Parzynski CS, et al. State mandated public reporting and outcomes of percutaneous coronary intervention in the United States. Am J Cardiol 2015;115(11):1494–501.

63. Joynt KE, Blumenthal DM, Orav EJ, et al. Association of public reporting for percutaneous coronary intervention with utilization and outcomes among Medicare beneficiaries with acute myocardial infarction. JAMA 2012;308(14):1460–8.

64. Apolito RA, Greenberg MA, Menegus MA, et al. Impact of the New York State Cardiac Surgery and Percutaneous Coronary Intervention Reporting System on the management of patients with acute myocardial infarction complicated by cardiogenic shock. Am Heart J 2008;155(2):267–73.

65. Waldo SW, McCabe JM, O'Brien C, et al. Association between public reporting of outcomes with procedural management and mortality for patients with acute myocardial infarction. J Am Coll Cardiol 2015;65(11):1119–26.

66. Fernandez G, Narins CR, Bruckel J, et al. Patient and Physician Perspectives on Public Reporting of Mortality Ratings for Percutaneous Coronary Intervention in New York State. Circ Cardiovasc Qual Outcomes 2017;10(9):e003511.

67. Blumenthal DM, Valsdottir LR, Zhao Y, et al. A survey of interventional cardiologists' attitudes and beliefs about public reporting of percutaneous coronary intervention. JAMA Cardiol 2018;3(7):629–34.

68. Boyden TF, Joynt KE, McCoy L, et al. Collaborative quality improvement vs public reporting for percutaneous coronary intervention: A comparison of percutaneous coronary intervention in New York vs Michigan. Am Heart J 2015;170(6):1227–33.

69. Wadhera RK, Joynt Maddox KE, Yeh RW, et al. Public reporting of percutaneous coronary intervention outcomes: moving beyond the status quo. JAMA Cardiol 2018;3(7):635–40.

Development of ST-elevation Myocardial Infarction Programs in Developing Countries
Global Challenges and Solutions

Roopa Salwan, MD, DM (Cardiology), MHCD 2012 HBS[a],
Ashok Seth, FRCP, FACC, MSCAI, FESC, FAPSIC, DSc[b],*

KEYWORDS

- Cardiovascular disease (CVD) • ST-elevation myocardial infarction (STEMI)
- Ischemic heart disease • Primary percutaneous coronary intervention (PPCI)
- Fibrinolytic therapy (FT) • Emergency medical system (EMS)

KEY POINTS

- STEMI management is time sensitive, early diagnosis and timely reperfusion by PPCI or Fibrinolytic therapy and pharmaco-invasive approach reduces morbidity and mortality.
- In developed countries, Regional system of STEMI care that integrate EMS, non PCI hospitals and PPCI hospitals have been shown to increase the number of patients with timely access to reperfusion therapy.
- LMIC have a high burden of STEMI in a younger population. With limited resources and a fragmented healthcare system there is an implementation gap of established therapies.
- Improvement in STEMI care is a key opportunity to reduce death and disability in this vulnerable, young population.
- Healthcare systems in LMIC can benefit by understanding various approaches used to create STEMI networks in developed countries over the last two decades to design care that is affordable, sustainable and scalable.

INTRODUCTION

Cardiovascular disease (CVD) continues to be the leading cause of death worldwide; approximately 80% of CVD deaths occur in low-income and middle-income countries (LMICs), and 40% of these are premature resulting in approximately 3 million ST-elevation myocardial infarction (STEMI) case each year.[1,2] The epidemiologic transition to a high burden of ischemic heart disease (IHD) has happened with greater rapidity in LMICs than in high-income countries (HICs). The lifestyle and environment exposures associated with globalization and urbanization have increased cardiovascular risk in the middle-income and lower-income strata. Coupled with a greater population growth in LMIC, the absolute number of individuals with premature IHD has increased substantially. Despite a lower prevalence of traditionally recognized risk factors in LMICs, higher event rates are observed compared with HICs, partially because the populations of these countries have less access to preventive and equitable health care systems.[3] Not only

---

Conflict of Interest: No conflict of Interest to disclose.
[a] Max Super Speciality Hospital, Saket, New Delhi 110017, India; [b] Fortis Escorts Heart Institute, Okhla Road, New Delhi 110025, India
* Corresponding author.
E-mail address: ashok.seth@fortishealthcare.com

does the inability to afford treatment of acute illnesses and subsequent follow-up make it difficult survive acute but also many fall into poverty each year due to out-of-pocket treatment expenses.

Health care essentially is a process of applying the best available medical knowledge—both research and clinical—to solve patients' health problems. The technological capability to do extraordinary things for patients has increased, as has patient demand, in a setting of constrained resources and expensive health care of variable quality. It is relevant to focus on the design and management of the processes and organizations that enable them to deliver proved medical treatments more efficiently and effectively.

CLINICAL BACKGROUND

The identification of thrombus in an occluded coronary artery of patients with STEMI in the early 1970s was followed by the development of fibrinolytic therapy (FT)[4,5] and a few years later by primary angioplasty to restore flow in the occluded artery.[6,7] This was followed by several randomized trials and meta-analyses that demonstrated that primary percutaneous coronary intervention (PPCI),[8] when performed in a timely manner by experienced operators, improves infarct artery patency and is associated with improved survival, lower rates of stroke, recurrent myocardial infarction (MI), and ischemia compared with FT. Also came the understanding of a direct relationship between symptom duration, infarct size, and mortality. STEMI management is time sensitive—time is muscle; delays in treatment were associated with worse outcomes irrespective of the reperfusion therapy used. PPCI is the preferred but not the only reperfusion strategy. For non–percutaneous coronary intervention (PCI)-capable hospitals, where transfer times exceeded 120 minutes, a pharmacoinvasive strategy of fibrinolysis combined with rescue PCI (in cases of failed fibrinolysis) or routine early PCI (in cases of successful fibrinolysis) is effective and safe.[9] FT is widely available and is the mainstay of treatment around the globe. The emphasis has shifted away from the choice of therapy toward ensuring that all eligible patients receive therapy efficiently and timely manner. It also has moved away from the concept of a stand-alone single hospital toward more community or region-based management strategy.

American College of Cardiology/American Heart Association (AHA) and European Society of Cardiology (ESC) STEMI[10,11] guidelines recommend (class 1 recommendation, level of evidence B) that all communities create and maintain a regional system of STEMI care that includes assessment and continuous quality improvement of emergency medical services (EMS) and hospital-based activities (Fig. 1).

1. To offer PPCI to the maximum proportion of patients within the recommended time spans
2. To provide optimal care for STEMI patients in the prehospital setting, including rapid and accurate diagnosis and preactivation of the cardiac catheterization laboratory
3. Initiation of pharmacologic reperfusion therapy (FT) if PPCI cannot be offered in a timely fashion
4. To increase the proportion of patients receiving timely PPCI by bypassing closer hospitals without interventional facilities

To narrow the gap between evidence and clinical practice for the community, a rigorous approach has been applied over the past 2 decades. Cardiovascular registries were established, which gave a glimpse of the changing landscape by providing clinicians with reliable data, which thy could use to improve their practice. Registries served as learning networks that set benchmarks and drove quality improvements. Sharing of data reduced variations in practice and translated into improvements in patient outcomes. Registries allow organic growth of studies evaluating process of care and outcomes and help define lacunae in care to facilitate the development and delivery of tools to overcome these lacunae. Quality improvement evolves from individual centers to collaborations at the regional level and then national level (Fig. 2).

The Global Registry of Acute Coronary Events was an international observational registry of patients with acute coronary syndromes (ACSs) between April 1999 and June 2006. It included 10,954 patients with STEMI; during this period, there was a significant increase in the use of PPCI from 15% to 44%, while use of FT decreased from 41% to 16%. The median time to fibrinolysis was reduced from 40 minutes to 34 minutes and mortality reduced from 6.9% to 5.7%; however, significant number of patients had treatment delay—42% of patients receiving PPCI had door-to-balloon (D2B) times greater than 90 minutes and 52% of patients receiving fibrinolysis had door-to-needle (D2N) times exceeding 30 minutes and 33% of patients still did not receive reperfusion therapy. Factors related with no reperfusion were prior heart failure, age greater than 75 years, prior MI, prior

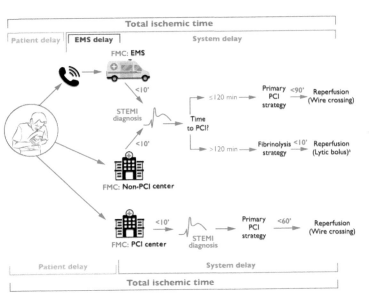

Fig. 1. Maximum target times according to reperfusion strategy selection in patients presenting via EMS or in a non-PCI center. STEMI diagnosis is the time 0 for the strategy clock. The decision for choosing reperfusion strategy in patients presenting via EMS (out-of-hospital setting) or in a non-PCI center is based on the estimated time from STEMI diagnosis to PCI-mediated reperfusion. Target times from STEMI diagnosis represent the maximum time to do specific interventions. ESC STEMI guidelines 2017. [a] Patients with fibrinolysis should be transferred to a PCI centre immediately after administration of the lytic bolus. (*From* European Heart Journal, Volume 39, Issue 2, 07 January 2018, Pages 119–177 [https://academic.oup.com/eurheartj/article/39/2/119/4095042]).

coronary artery bypass graft, female sex, diabetes, and delay from symptom onset to hospital arrival (patient delay).[12]

The National Registry of Myocardial Infarction was a prospective US registry, running from 1990 to 2006, which collected data on reperfusion therapy, including D2N and D2B times of 1,374,232 patients with STEMI. Over these years, use of fibrinolysis reduced from 52.5% to 27.6% and PPCI increased from 2.6% to 43.4%. The proportion of STEMI patients eligible for but not receiving reperfusion therapy decreased significantly, from 44.9% in 1990 to 28.1% in 2006 (P<.001). There were significant reductions in D2N time, from 59 minutes to 29 minutes, and a decrease in in-hospital mortality for patients treated with fibrinolysis, from 7.0% to 6.0%. Among patients who were treated with primary PCI, the overall D2B time decreased from 120 minutes in 1994 to 87 minutes in 2006, with a decrease in in-hospital mortality from 8.6% in 1994 to 3.3% in 2006.[13] D2B was a composite of presentation to electrocardiogram (ECG), ECG to treatment decision, treatment decision to transfer initiation, and transport time and catheterization laboratory receiving time to restoration of flow Several organizational barriers—delays in triage, evaluation, and diagnosis and limited staffing during off-hours, which may affect the overall efficacy of primary PCI—were identified. As the momentum for primary

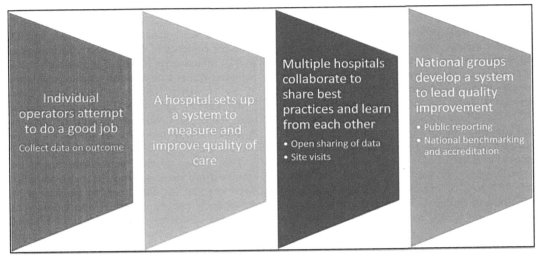

Fig. 2. Stages of quality improvement.

PCI grew, systems to improved process-of-care were needed more than ever.

Evolution of ST-elevation Myocardial Infarction Networks in Europe

Europe has a highly sophisticated ambulance system; landmark trials established that interhospital transfer for primary PCI was better than fibrinolysis. This was reflected in the ESC guidelines and STEMI systems of care in Europe, which are well established, primary PCI being the preferred reperfusion strategy for a majority of STEMI patients. There is close cooperation between EMS and tertiary centers and community hospitals.[14–16]

In France, the Service d'Aide Médicale Urgente network was started in 1995, with a unique nationwide call number to optimize coordination between ambulances, non-PCI, and primary PCI centers. Physicians staffed ambulances enabled early initiation of treatment and prehospital fibrinolysis. Since 2005, regional networks have been implemented in most French regions, with most patients now admitted or transferred to hospitals with catheterization laboratories. Patients presenting to smaller hospitals are transferred immediately to tertiary care centers using mobile intensive care units.

Every 5 years since 1995 [USIK 1995, Management of acute myocardial infarction in intensive care units in 1995: a nationwide French survey, USIC (Unite de Soins Intensifs Coronaires) 2000, FAST-MI (French Registry of Acute ST-Elevation or non-ST-elevation Myocardial Infarction) 2005, FAST-MI 2010 and FAST-MI 2015] a 1-month, nationwide survey of patients with AMI has been performed, with the aim of providing cardiologists and health authorities national and regional data on acute MI (AMI) management and outcomes. This registry included at least 60% of all institutions taking care of patients with AMI, and the patients were followed for at least 1 year. In 2005%, 29% were treated with thrombolytics before transfer (18% prehospital); in-hospital mortality rates were 4.3% for thrombolysis and 5.0% for PPCI. There was no significant difference in 5-year survival rates for STEMI patients as analyzed by reperfusion strategy—fibrinolysis (both prehospital and in-hospital combined) versus PPCI. In the 20 years, the use of primary PCI increased from 12% to 71%, in-hospital mortality was 2.8% in 2015, and 6-month mortality reduced significantly, from 17.2% to 6.9% in 2010 and to 5.3% in 2015.[17]

In England, from 2003 to 2011, the rate of PPCI increased from 46% to 94% as part of a National Health Service improvement program using cardiac networks to improve access and use of PPCI to improve survival. With this, 30-day mortality for STEMI fell by 31%, from 12.4% to 8.6%. In many regions, to optimize catheterization laboratory utilization, a rotational system between tertiary centers is arranged; whereas during the day times, all centers are available, and during night duty, limited active centers are available.

In Norway and other European countries, mountain terrain long transfer distances limit the ability to provide PPCI to patients in rural areas, prehospital FT followed by pharmacoinvasive strategy remains the cornerstone of treatment.[18]

Evolution of ST-elevation Myocardial Infarction Networks in the United States

The US health care landscape is diverse, with several catheterization laboratories in urban areas and paucity of laboratories in rural areas. Therefore, the requirements to establish networks differ in various regions.

The Minneapolis Heart Institute initiated one of the first regional interhospital transfer STEMI systems in the United States by developing a hub-and-spoke model, with 30 referral non-PCI hospitals in a 210-mile radius as spokes and a 24 × 7 PCI centers as a hub. The spoke hospitals were divided into 2 zones: zone 1, less than 60 miles, were direct transferred; and zone 2, 60 miles to 210 miles, received half-dose fibrinolytics and were transferred. They were able to show that rapid transfer of STEMI patients from community hospitals to a PCI center was safe and effective using a standardized protocol with an integrated transfer system. From March 2003 to November 2006, 1345 consecutive STEMI patients (78% transferred from non-PCI hospitals) were treated. The median first D2B time for patients in zone 1 was 95 minutes and as 120 minutes for zone 2. For this high-risk unselected patient population (cardiogenic shock, 12.3%; cardiac arrest, 10.8%; and elderly [≥80 years of age], 14.6%), in-hospital mortality was 4.2%, and median length of stay was 3 days, 30-day mortality of 4.9%, and 1-year mortality of 7.2% (5.7% cardiovascular).[19]

The success of this system was based on a standardized protocol and extensive training at each hospital for EMS, nursing personnel, and emergency department (ED) and primary care physicians. Each hospital had a level 1 MI toolkit that included a protocol checklist, transfer forms, clinical data form, standing orders, adjunctive medications, and laboratory supplies.

The clinical data form, ECG, and laboratory results were faxed to the PCI center cardiac catheterization laboratory. Transferred patients were taken directly to the cardiac catheterization laboratory for PCI without re-evaluation in the ED. Backup protocols were in place for anticipated delays (such as inclement weather): zone 1, half-dose fibrinolytic and facilitated PCI; and zone 2, full dose fibrinolytic.

Shortly after the creation of the MHI STEMI network, Los Angeles County began formulating its unique network of STEMI receiving centers—hospitals that provide primary PCI around the clock and also accept STEMI patients even when the hospital's ED is on diversion because of overcrowding. Los Angeles had multiple hubs strategically located and they focused on a prehospital triage model: prehospital ECG transmission with immediate frontline physician review to facilitate direct admission to the catheterization laboratory bypassing the ED.[20]

The Regional Approach to Cardiovascular Emergencies investigators who were able to develop a statewide STEMI network system to include all 119 hospitals in North Carolina. Over an 18-month period, 6841 STEMI patients were enrolled, including 3907 who presented directly to 21 PCI hospitals and 2933 patients who were transferred from 98 non-PCI hospitals; a median D2B time of 59 minutes was achieved and the time from first door-to-device for patients transferred from a non-PCI for PCI improved to 103 minutes, with 39% of patients treated within 90 minutes.[21,22]

The Mayo Clinic also reported their implementation of a protocol to coordinate systems of care for a PCI center and 28 regional hospitals within 150 miles across 3 states and was able to increase the number of STEMI patient with timely access to PPCI.[23]

The purpose of such networks was to increase the rates of reperfusion therapy, to maintain the lowest possible D2B and D2N times, and ultimately to reduce associated morbidity and mortality. The demonstration of benefits associated with these networks was consistent.

Progress in the United States and Europe did not occur overnight. It was a result of steadfast determination and focused directives from cardiology societies and working groups, which resulted in step-by-step and incremental system improvements.

In 2007, there was great variation in the type of reperfusion: 30% eligible patients did not receive reperfusion, 70% of fibrinolytic ineligible patients did not receive PPCI, 50% patients undergoing FT had D2N less than 30 minutes, and 40%

patients undergoing PPCI had D2B less than 90 minutes. There clearly was a need to set up networks of care to overcome real-world obstacles, reduce treatment delays, and increase the proportion of patients benefiting from reperfusion. At that time, 76% STEMI patients arrived at the hospital via self-transport; primary care and specialist physicians worked in isolation, perceiving a loss of patient and prestige on referring to a PCI center; and EMS was fragmented. It was realized that non-PCI hospitals were pivotal in increasing timely access to reperfusion and developing them as STEMI referral hospitals with protocols for care and transfer helped integrate them in the system.

The AHA held a summit, "Development of Systems of Care for ST-Elevation Myocardial Infarction Patients," that brought together stakeholders in STEMI care: patients, physicians, nurses, EMS and ED personnel, hospital administrators, payers, and outcomes experts.[24,25] The perspective they gave enabled the AHA to launch the largest national effort to organize STEMI care Mission: Lifeline, and later the STEMI Systems Accelerator project that involved 23,809 patients treated at 484 hospitals and 1253 EMS agencies in 16 regions. By shifting focus from hospital to system time (first medical contact to device time), they were able to improve not only reperfusion time but also survival (Box 1).[26]

IMPLEMENTATION GAPS IN LOW-INCOME AND MIDDLE-INCOME COUNTRIES

The implementation of guideline-based treatment has improved the outcomes of STEMI in HICs whereas there is a huge implementation gap of established therapies in LMICs. Improving the availability and delivery of proved, effective therapies in diverse socioeconomic settings and populations is critical to reducing mortality burden in LMIC. The United Nations sustainable development goals include a target to reduce premature mortality from noncommunicable diseases by one-third by 2030.

Major inequalities exist in the care of AMI in developed and developing countries. Quality of care is the main challenge to implementing treatment. The first health care providers are diverse in their expertise and understanding, often have dubious credentials, and have less knowledge about complex issues. Ambulance services are sparse or often nonexistent; doctors and nurses trained to deliver thrombolytic therapy, recognize and treat arrhythmia, or perform PPCI are few and scattered. The current

---

Box 1
Essentials for ST-elevation myocardial infarction systems of care

Single emergency number

EMS triage: Ambulances equipped with 12-lead ECGs and defibrillators, and staffed with physicians or well-trained paramedics to diagnose STEMI, or capable ECG telemetry. Protocols for direct transfer to Cath Lab

Interfacility transfer protocols, Door In - Door Out at non PCI Hospitals for the STEMI patient transferring out for Primary PCI, Fibrinolytic protocols if transfer time exceeds 120 min, followed transfer protocols for Pharmacoinvasive approach

Emergency Department protocols Direct telephone access to the Cath lab: single Call to activate the system

Cardiac CATH Lab teams protocols: PCI capable facilities that are open 24 hours a day and 7 days a week

Cardiologist or intensive care specialist as a network leader

Comprehensive real-time data prospective data collection, prompt, consistent feedback, quality assurance, Involvement of healthcare authorities

Public information campaigns Community engagement, cultural relevance, appropriateness

Prospective registry

---

unstructured and highly inefficient system of management in most LMICs means that the gains from revascularization therapies as seen in developed countries seldom can be achieved in LMIC. Such a system puts the onus on patients (and their families) to reach the right hospital within the right time frame and with adequate finances for out-of-pocket payments. National benchmarks and registries to track the changing practices are lacking. As a result, acute mortality and long-term outcomes are not comparable to that achieved in developed countries. Thus, improving access to primary PCI and the pharmacoinvasive approach re important priorities for LMICs and offers a key opportunity for their health care systems to reduce the burden of death and disability in a young population.

It is important to understand health-seeking pathways of patients: mere awareness does not result in quick and appropriate action; patients often wait until their condition deteriorates. The first responders often are unregistered practitioners of alternative medicine—ayurveda, Unani, Siddha, homeopathy—they are important

from public health perspective. Lack of awareness of the importance of early treatment and perceived economic barriers lead patients to treatment shopping and delays. Decision to shop for advice is based on mistrust and lack of confidence on the of the provider coupled with denial and nonacceptance of diagnosis.[27] The solution lies in the public and private hospitals that must work as equal partners, supporting and complementing each other; there must be an efficient referral between providers of different levels of care.

Advancements in telecommunication and the Internet can go a long way toward redefining appropriate care pathways in many LMICs. Telemedicine offers a cost-effective method of creating large-scale population-based STEMI networks of care that utilize local synergies to overcome vast infrastructure deficits. Telemedicine is used as a foundation pillar to initiate an optimal strategy for global AMI management. ECG is the single investigation required to diagnose STEMI in a patient with chest pain. The median accuracy of ECG interpretation has been found to be 42.0% for medical students, 55.8% for residents, 68.5% for practicing physicians, and 74.9% for cardiologists. Accuracy increased with training and specialization. Hospitalization for triage and risk stratification of chest pain is expensive and difficult. Poorly managed care or missed diagnosis results in expensive and avoidable complications. Beneficiaries of publicly funded health programs are less likely to receive high-quality care. Telemedicine has emerged as a cost-effective technology to improve access and accuracy to diagnose STEMI (ECG interpretation) and facilitate triage to closest treatment center (tele-consultation).

Lumen America Telemedicine Infarct Network (LATIN) provides the world's first and comprehensive population-based AMI strategy that uses telemedicine to provide global AMI care and it may be a revolutionary start to bridging the gap between the disparate levels of AMI care. Between 2013 and 2019, LATIN covered an area populated by 100 million people in remote areas of Argentina, Brazil, Colombia, and Mexico. The network included a hub-and-spoke model; telemedicine devices were located strategically in ambulances; remote locations, in primary clinics, private nursing homes, General Practitioner clinics, patients presenting with chest pain undergo ECG that is analysed by telemedicine experts and are triaged to fibrinolytic therapy, pharmacoinvasive management, and primary PCI. Of 780,234 patients screened at 313 centers, or spokes, in remote locations, 1.1% were diagnosed with STEMI. Of the diagnosed patients, 46.1% were transferred to 1 of 47 hubs, and, of these, 78% underwent reperfusion therapy with PCI. Time to telemedicine diagnosis was 3.5 minutes, mean D2B time was 48 minutes, and the STEMI mortality rate was 5.2%.[28]

On a smaller scale, the authors demonstrated the ability of electronic intensive care unit (eICU) to reduce mortality in STEMI patients in resource limited areas. The eICU was established in a hill town, where the nearest health care facility was 10 hours away by surface transport, with remote monitoring from a heart command center in Delhi. The eICU had complete access to patients' vitals and treatment. Patients presenting with chest pain and ST elevation were treated with fibrinolytic therapy within 30 minutes of arrival. With this system in place, the in-hospital mortality was reduced from 16.4% to 4.8%.[29]

ST-ELEVATION MYOCARDIAL INFARCTION NETWORK IN CHINA

The health care delivery is state controlled and, over the past 2 decades, China first conducted a retrospective study on the state of care delivery and going ahead has put in place a 10-year plan of sequential development of networks of care.

The China Patient-Centered Evaluative Assessment of Cardiac Events–Retrospective Acute Myocardial Infarction Study was a nationally representative study, on the clinical profile, management, and outcome of 13,815 STEMI patients in the decade 2001 to 2011. The estimated national rates of hospital admission for STEMI per 100,000 people increased from 3.5 in 2001, to 7.9 in 2006, and to 15.4 in 2011; (P<.0001). The rate of primary PCI increased from 10.1% to 28.1% and the use of FT reduced from 44.1% to 27%; the percentage of patients who did not receive reperfusion therapy did not change 45.3% in 2001 versus 44.8% in 2011. The risk of death, treatment withdrawal, and complications did not change over time; mortality was 8.4% in 2001 and 7% in 2011. An increased prevalence of coronary risk factors, persistent delays in admission to hospital, increasing use of procedures and tests, relatively long hospital stays, and gaps in quality of care with the underuse of guideline-recommended therapies and the use of therapies of unknown effectiveness were identified. Such large-scale registries focusing on clinical pathways strengthened the understanding of the need to set up regional emergency care networks.[30]

The China STEMI Care Project is a 10-year project launched in 18 provinces, to improve reperfusion therapy, with protocol for pharmacoinvasive therapy in non-PCI hospitals. It is being developed in 3 phases: phase 1, in-hospital process optimization of primary PCI hospitals; phase 2, STEMI care network construction with adjacent non-PPCI hospitals and EMS; phase 3, whole-fcity STEMI care network construction with chest pain centers. Central to these processes is systematic data collection, assessment of quality of care, and patient outcome, with continuous data-driven improvement in quality of care.[31]

ST-ELEVATION MYOCARDIAL INFARCTION NETWORK IN INDIA
The CREATE Registry

Treatment and outcomes of acute coronary syndromes in India (CREATE) was a prospective registry (2001–2005) of 20,468 patients in 89 centers from 50 cities in India. Patients of AMI with definite ECG changes (whether elevated ST [STEMI] or non-STEMI or unstable angina) or had suspected MI without ECG changes but with prior evidence of IHD were studied; 60.6% had STEMI, mean age of these patients was 56.3 years, and 52.5% patients were from lower middle and 19.6% from poor social classes. The median time from symptoms to hospital was 360 minutes, thrombolytic therapy was used in 58.5% (96.3% was streptokinase)and PPCI in 8%. The 30-day outcomes for patients with STEMI were death (8.6%), reinfarction (2.3%), and stroke (0.7%). Rich patients were more likely to get thrombolytic therapy compared with poor patients (60.6% vs 52.3%, respectively).[32]

Kerala Acute Coronary Syndrome Registry

Kerala, the most advanced Indian state in epidemiologic transition, has had to pivot its health care delivery system to face the burden of non-communicable diseases. The overall age-adjusted prevalence of definite coronary artery disease (CAD) has been found to be 3.5% (men, 4.8%, and women, 2.6%).

In a prospective registry of 25,748 consecutive ACS admissions from 2007 to 2009 in 125 hospitals in Kerala, 37% of patients had STEMI; thrombolytics were used in 41% of STEMI and PPCI in 12.8%; and in-hospital mortality was 8.2%.[33] Quality improvement is an unending cycle wherein high-quality data are collected and used to identify gaps in care processes; quality improvement efforts then are developed to bridge these gaps, with resultant improvements in care. The lessons learnt then are shared across the network. The registry has been followed-up by a program for quality improvement in the entire state. The STEMI network is built on evidence and on guideline recommendations to enhance the speed and delivery of reperfusion therapy to all eligible patients, led by inspired and respected local champions. It is adapted to local conditions, is simple to follow, has acceptance from all stakeholders, and includes continuous data surveillance and feedback linked with quality improvement and adaptability to new knowledge.[34]

In a recent publication on procedural volume and outcome after PPCI in STEMI, from June 2013 to March 2016, 5560 consecutive patients were studied in 42 hospitals: low volume (<100 PPCI per year), 57.2%; medium volume (100–199 PPCI), 19%; and high volume (>200 PPCI), 23.8%. Total ischemic time (median) was 3.5 hours among low-volume hospitals, 3.8 hours in medium-volume hospitals, and 4.16 hours in high-volume hospitals. Patients classified as living in poverty preferentially accessed high-volume hospitals, many of whom were offering government-sponsored health insurance, possibly bypassing nearby low-volume hospitals. The observed 1-year mortality rates were 6.5%, 3.4%, and 8.6% at low-volume, medium-volume, and high-volume hospitals, respectively ($P<.01$). LMICs, like India, may have a unique nonlinear relationship between institutional-level PPCI volumes and outcomes, with high-volume hospitals having the highest 1-year mortality rates STEMI infarction. Quality-improvement initiatives should at first focus on the relatively few high-volume hospitals. Process-of-care metrics, like timeliness of reperfusion and PPCI procedural characteristics, may be the key to improving STEMI outcomes in India rather than institutional-level PPCI volumes.[35]

Tamil Nadu ST-elevation Myocardial Infarctions Program

The Tamil Nadu STEMI Program was a multicenter, prospective, observational study conducted in Tamil Nadu, India, that implemented a hub-and-spoke model of care (linking 35 spoke health centers to the 4 large PCI hub hospitals), leveraging developments in public health insurance schemes, EMS, and health information technology to enhance patient access to care. In this project, 2420 patients with STEMI were evaluated in a pre-implementation (2012–2013; n = 898)/post-implementation (2013–2014; n = 1522) design. This integrated system greatly improved process measures from pre-implementation to post-implementation, such as fibrinolysis to PCI time (39.2 vs 17.3 hours, respectively; $P = .003$), performance of coronary angiography (35.0% vs 60.8%, respectively;

$P<.0001$), and primary PCI use (21.8% vs 40.7%, respectively; $P<.0001$); there was no change in D2B time for PPCI (100 min vs 105 min, respectively). The use of a pharmacoinvasive strategy also increased (13.1% vs 20.1%, respectively; $P<.0001$), particularly among spoke hospital patients (2.5% vs 28.2%, respectively; $P<.0001$). In-hospital mortality was not different (52 [5.8%] vs 85 [5.6%], respectively; $P = .83$), with a significantly lower 1-year mortality (17.6% vs 14.2%, respectively). In-hospital mortality was significantly lower in the hub hospital patients compared with patients initially evaluated at the spoke health care centers during the pre-implementation phase (15 [3.6%] vs 37 [7.6%], respectively; $P = .01$), but this difference was not present during the post-implementation phase (49 [5.1%] vs 36 [6.3%], respectively; $P = .42$). Standalone fibrinolysis was reduced from 53.6% to 29.4% in the hubs and 77.1% to 46.3% in the spoke centers.[36]

The high mortality rate at 1 year (17.2% vs 14.2%, respectively) needs to be analyzed in detail; noncompliance with dual-antiplatelet therapy and suboptimal risk factor control are important components of high event rates on follow-up. Appropriateness of care to ensure long-term favorable outcomes has to be structured in planning of care. The processes are in place and the journey of quality improvement has to follow the cycles of learning and implementation.

Himachal Pradesh ST-elevation Myocardial Infarction Registry

The Himachal Pradesh STEMI registry is a collaborative effort involving 33 hospitals in the hilly state of Himachal Pradesh, initiated in 2012. In the first report of 5182 patients, 45% were STEMI cases and 83% were from rural areas; mean time to presentation was 13 hours. Over a 6-year follow up, the reperfusion rate increased from approximately 21% to 42%, primarily because of increase in PCI rate from 2.2% to 21.9%, while the thrombolytic therapy rate remained at 35%, due to delayed presentation; significant decline in the in-hospital mortality rates from 9.0% to 6.1% has been seen.[37]

THE WAY FORWARD

A white paper on appropriate resource and infrastructure management of STEMI in LMIC recently has been published to provide guidelines to frontline clinicians and government agencies to enable the improvement in STEMI care.[38] It describes a 5-tiered approach to setting up a STEMI network. In any region, there are 5 levels of care providers:

> Level 1 is a general practitioner or a primary health center, without ability to record ECG.
> Level 2 is a clinic or community health center with ability to record ECG.
> Level 3 is a center equipped to diagnose STEMI and deliver thrombolytic therapy.
> Level 4 is a center equipped to perform PPCI after diagnosis of STEMI, with a catheterization laboratory in working hours.
> Level 5 is a 24 × 7 catheterization laboratory and trained personnel to diagnose and treat STEMI by PPCI.

This document identifies the knowledge and implementation gaps in LMIC.[38] The point of first medical contact is crucial to diagnosis, administration of basic treatment, and referral to the closest center that can provide appropriate care. Accreditation of STEMI care centers by existing bodies, International Standards Organization 9000, Joint Commission on Accreditation of Healthcare Organizations, and National Accreditation Board of Hospitals and Healthcare Providers, for level of care provided is important to enable the community to know the care available and as an impetus for the center to maintain standards of care. Each region should map its available facilities and develop formal referral channels to help patients navigate the health care system efficiently.

It also recommends the participation of the government in providing social insurance, setting up ambulance networks, legislation to accredit STEMI hospitals and EMS, and developing shared ambulance networks and optimal utilization of technology to increase reach to the population. The creation of data collection tools and analytics is an integral part of the care system that will enable outcome measurement and help quality improvement. Postdischarge care and follow-up are vital parts of the process.

In a landmark decision, stents were placed on the National List of Essential Medications in July 2016 by the health ministry of India. Then, in 2017, India's National Pharmaceutical and Pricing Authority made a landmark decision to fix price ceilings for coronary stents. These decisions have increased the procedures being done.

Public–private partnership (PPP) is an important way forward for health care in developing countries Given the respective strengths and weaknesses, neither the public sector nor private sector alone is in the best interest of the health system. Delivery of health care is all about patient outcome—both public and private hospitals need to be accountable. The services provided have to be measurable. Government continues to play a critical role but needs to play a new role, to continue public sector reform and strengthen ability to deliver services and institution capacity. The public health system is not driven by policy and lacks continuity. Also, there no organization to manage PPP and private sectors; PPP is not the same as privatization.

The private health care sector has grown in the past 3 decades and is playing an important role in the delivery of health care. Larger hospital groups have national and international accreditation and strive to be accountable and be patient outcome driven.

The private sector has improved access, efficiency, and accountability and helped imbibe best practices. There are concerns, however, toward unbridled commercial behavior of the private sector and cultural antipathy toward private sector.

The way ahead is a collaboration with transparent terms and conditions, partner obligations, performance indicators, and overall health objectives. Partnerships entail relative equality between partners, mutual commitment to health objectives, shared decision making and accountability, and equitable returns/outcomes. It may take time for systems in LMIC to mature but efforts are underway because it is the only way forward.

SUMMARY

The developing world faces the highest burden of disease, with limited infrastructure and paucity of skilled manpower. All stakeholders have to come together to optimally utilize resources and invest in integrating existing resources to improve treatment and outcomes in this young population. STEMI care networks aim to provide high-quality care that is patient-centered, safe, effective, and timely, with a reduction in disparities of health care delivery across economic, educational, racial/ethnic, and geographic boundaries. Basic structure provides for early diagnosis, rapid patient transfer for optimal door-to-reperfusion time, and well-integrated first responders and emergency, ambulance, and in-hospital teams. Data collection and feedback in registries will provide the opportunity to detect problems within the respective systems of care and grow the program organically. Engaging with all stakeholders is important—the discussion has to move beyond cardiologists. Collaboration between public and private hospitals and policy that invests in these collaborations and works on strengths would enable delivery of optimal care to a larger population.

CLINICS CARE POINTS

- Early diagnosis and triage to appropriate care – the first responders are often practitioners of alternative medicine, integrating them in the chain of care is important for increasing uptake of treatment, building trust.

- Telemedicine has emerged as a cost effective technology to improve access, accuracy to diagnose STEMI and triage to nearest reperfusion capable hospital.

- Standardised protocols for STEMI care, with clearly defined roles and responsibilities, should be prepared in each hospital according to the manpower and infrastructure available, followed by integration of hospitals in a region with clear mapping of PPCI and non PCI hospitals. Non PCI hospitals are pivotal in increasing access to reperfusion.

- Data collection and feedback reduces variations in practice and improves patient outcome.

- Policy that makes care affordable, promotes cooperation within existing facilities, engages with all stakeholders with clear roadmap for sustainable improvement.

REFERENCES

1. Prabhakaran D, Anand S, Watkins D, et al. Cardiovascular, respiratory, and related disorders: key messages from disease control priorities, 3rd edition. Lancet 2018;391(10126):1224–36.
2. Vedanthan R, Seligman B, Fuster V. Global perspective on acute coronary syndrome: a burden on the young and poor. Circ Res 2014;114:1959–75.
3. Yusuf S, Rangarajan S, Teo K, et al. Cardiovascular risk and events in 17 low-, middle-, and high-income countries. N Engl J Med 2014;371(9): 818–27.
4. Gruppo Italiano per lo Studio della Streptochinasi nell'Infarto Miocardico (GISSI). Effectiveness of intravenous thrombolytic treatment in acute myocardial infarction. Lancet 1986;1(8478):397–402.
5. ISIS-2 (Second International Study of Infarct Survival) Collaborative Group. Randomised trial of intravenous streptokinase, oral aspirin, both, or neither among 17,187 cases of suspected acute myocardial infarction: ISIS-2. Lancet 1988;2:349–60.
6. Hartzler GO, Rutherford BD, McConahay DR, et al. Percutaneous transluminal coronary angioplasty with and without thrombolytic therapy for treatment of acute myocardial infarction. Am Heart J 1983;106:965–73.
7. Zijlstra F, de Boer MJ, Hoorntje JC, et al. A comparison of immediate coronary angioplasty with intravenous streptokinase in acute myocardial infarction. N Engl J Med 1993;328:680–4.
8. Keeley EC, Boura JA, Grines CL. Primary angioplasty versus intravenous thrombolytic therapy for acute myocardial infarction: A quantitative review of 23 randomised trials. Lancet 2003;361:13–20.
9. Armstrong PW, Gershlick AH, Goldstein P, et al. Kurt Huber, Stefan Grajek, Claudio Fresco, Erich Bluhmki, Anne Regelin, Katleen Vandenberghe, Kris Bogaerts, and Frans Van de Werf, for the STREAM Investigative Team. Fibrinolysis or Primary PCI in ST-Segment Elevation Myocardial Infarction. N Engl J Med 2013;368:1379–87.
10. O'Gara PT, Kushner FG, Ascheim DD, et al. 2013 ACCF/AHA guideline for the management of ST-elevation myocardial infarction: executive summary: A report of the American College of Cardiology Foundation/American Heart Association Task Force on Practice Guidelines. Circulation 2013;127:529–55.
11. Ibanez B, James S, Agewall S, et al. 2017 ESC Guidelines for the management of acute myocardial infarction in patients presenting with ST-segment elevation: The Task Force for the management of acute myocardial infarction in patients presenting with ST-segment elevation of the European Society of Cardiology (ESC). Eur Heart J 2018;39(2):119–77. https://doi.org/10.1093/eurheartj/ehx393.
12. Eagle KA, Goodman SG, Avezum A, et al. Practice variation and missed opportunities for reperfusion in ST-segment-elevation myocardial infarction: findings from the Global Registry of Acute Coronary Events (GRACE). Lancet 2002;359:373–7.
13. Nallamothu BK, Bates ER, Herrin J, et al, for the NRMI Investigators. Times to Treatment in Transfer Patients Undergoing Primary Percutaneous Coronary Intervention in the United States National Registry of Myocardial Infarction (NRMI)-3/4 Analysis. Circulation 2005;111:761–7.
14. Vermeer F, Oude Ophuis AJ, van den Berg EJ, et al. Prospective randomised comparison between thrombolysis, rescue PTCA, and primary PTCA in patients with extensive myocardial infarction admitted to a hospital without PTCA facilities: a safety and feasibility study. Heart 1999;82:426–31.
15. Widimský P, Budesinský T, Vorác D, et al. Long distance transport for primary angioplasty vs immediate

thrombolysis in acute myocardial infarction: final results of the randomized national multicentre trial — PRAGUE-2. Eur Heart J 2003;24:94–104.

16. Zijlstra F. Angioplasty vs thrombolysis for acute myocardial infarction: a quantitative overview of the effects of interhospital transportation. Eur Heart J 2003;24:21–3.

17. Hanssen M, Cottin Y, Khalife K, et al, for the FAST-MI 2010 investigators. French Registry on Acute ST-elevation and non ST-elevation Myocardial Infarction 2010. FAST-MI 2010. Heart 2012;98:699e705.

18. Bøhmer E, Hoffmann P, Abdelnoor M, et al. Efficacy and safety of immediate angioplasty versus ischemia-guided management after thrombolysis in acute myocardial infarction in areas with very long transfer distances results of the NORDISTEMI (NORwegian study on DIstrict treatment of ST-elevation myocardial infarction). J Am Coll Cardiol 2010;55(2):102–10.

19. Henry TD, Sharkey SW, Burke MN, et al. A regional system to provide timely access to percutaneous coronary intervention for ST-elevation myocardial infarction. Circulation 2007;116:721–8.

20. Rokos IC, French WJ, Koenig WJ, et al. Integration of pre-hospital electrocardiograms and ST-elevation myocardial infarction receiving (SRC) networks: impact on door-to-balloon times across 10 independent regions. JACC Cardiovasc Interv 2009;2:339–46.

21. Jollis JG, Roettig ML, Aluko AO, et al. Reperfusion of Acute Myocardial Infarction in North Carolina Emergency Departments (RACE) Investigators. Implementation of a statewide system for coronary reperfusion for ST-segment elevation myocardial infarction. JAMA 2007;298:2371–80.

22. Jollis JG, Al-Khalidi HR, Monk L, et al, on behalf of the RACE Investigators. Expansion of a regional ST-segment elevation myocardial infarction system to an entire state. Circulation 2012;126:189–95.

23. Ting HH, Rihal CS, Gersh BJ, et al. Regional systems of care to optimize timeliness of reperfusion therapy for ST-elevation myocardial infarction: the Mayo Clinic STEMI Protocol. Circulation 2007;116:729–36.

24. Jacobs AK, Antman EM, Ellrodt G, et al. American Heart Association's Acute Myocardial Infarction Advisory Working Group. Recommendation to develop strategies to increase the number of ST-segment-elevation myocardial infarction patients with timely access to primary percutaneous coronary intervention. Circulation 2006;113:2152–63.

25. Jacobs AK, Antman EM, Faxon DP, et al. Development of systems of care for ST-elevation myocardial infarction patients: executive summary. Circulation 2007;116:217230.

26. Jollis JG, Al-Khalidi HR, Roettig ML, et al. STEMI Systems Accelerator Project. Regional systems of care demonstration project: American Heart Association Mission: Lifeline STEMI Systems Accelerator. Circulation 2016;134:365374.

27. Bhattacharya Chakravarty A, Rangan S, Dholakia Y, et al. Such a long journey: what health seeking pathways of patients with drug resistant tuberculosis in Mumbai tell us? PLoS One 2019;14:e0209924.

28. Mehta S, Botelho R, Rodriguez D, et al. A tale of two cities: STEMI interventions in developed and developing countries and the potential of telemedicine to reduce disparities in care. J Interv Cardiol 2014;27:155–66.

29. Gupta S, Dewan S, Kaushal A, et al. EICU reduces mortality in STEMI patients in resource limited areas. Glob Heart 2014;9(4):425–7.

30. Li J, Xi Li, Wang Q, et al. ST-segment elevation myocardial infarction in China from 2001 to 2011 (the China PEACE-Retrospective Acute Myocardial Infarction Study): A retrospective analysis of hospital data. Lancet 2015;385:441–51.

31. Zhang Y, Yu B, Han Y, et al. Protocol of the China ST-segment elevation myocardial infarction (STEMI) Care Project (CSCAP): A 10-year project to improve quality of care by building up a regional STEMI care network. BMJ Open 2019;9:e026362.

32. Xavier D, Pais P, Devereaux PJ, et al. CREATE Registry Investigators. Treatment and outcomes of acute coronary syndromes in India: A prospective analysis of registry data. Lancet 2008;371:1435–42.

33. Mohanan PP, Mathew R, Harikrishnan S, et al. Presentation, management, and outcomes of 25 748 acute coronary syndrome admissions in Kerala, India: results from the Kerala ACS Registry. Eur Heart J 2013;34:121–9.

34. Mathew A, Abdullakutty J, Sebastian P, et al. Population access to reperfusion services for ST-segment elevation myocardial infarction in Kerala, India. Indian Heart J 2017;69:S51–6.

35. Jabir A, Mathew A, Zheng Y, et al. Procedural Volume and Outcomes after Primary Percutaneous Coronary Intervention for ST-Segment–Elevation Myocardial Infarction in Kerala, India: Report of the Cardiological Society of India–Kerala Primary Percutaneous Coronary Intervention Registry. J Am Heart Assoc 2020;9:e014968.

36. Alexander T, Mullasari AS, Joseph G, et al. A system of care for patients with ST-segment elevation myocardial infarction in India: the Tamil Nadu-ST-Segment Elevation Myocardial Infarction Program. JAMA Cardiol 2017;2:498–505.

37. Negi PC, Merwaha R, Panday D, et al. Multicenter HP ACS Registry. Indian Heart J 2016;68:118–27.

38. Chandrashekhar Y, Alexander T, Mullasari A, et al. Resource and infrastructure-appropriate management of ST-segment elevation myocardial infarction in low- and middle-income countries. Circulation 2020;141(24):2004–25.

Moving?

Make sure your subscription moves with you!

To notify us of your new address, find your **Clinics Account Number** (located on your mailing label above your name), and contact customer service at:

Email: journalscustomerservice-usa@elsevier.com

800-654-2452 (subscribers in the U.S. & Canada)
314-447-8871 (subscribers outside of the U.S. & Canada)

Fax number: 314-447-8029

Elsevier Health Sciences Division
Subscription Customer Service
3251 Riverport Lane
Maryland Heights, MO 63043

*To ensure uninterrupted delivery of your subscription, please notify us at least 4 weeks in advance of move.